EXPRESSIVE THERAPIES

Expressive Therapies

Edited by
CATHY A. MALCHIODI

Foreword by Shaun McNiff

THE GUILFORD PRESS
New York   London

© 2005 The Guilford Press
A Division of Guilford Publications, Inc.
72 Spring Street, New York, NY 10012
www.guilford.com

Printed in the United States of America

This book is printed on acid-free paper.

Last digit is print number: 9 8 7 6 5 4 3 2 1

Library of Congress Cataloging-in-Publication Data

Expressive therapies / edited by Cathy A. Malchiodi ; foreword by Shaun McNiff.
    p. cm.
  Includes bibliographical references and index.
  ISBN 1-59385-087-5 (hardcover : alk. paper)
  1. Arts—Therapeutic use. I. Malchiodi, Cathy A.
  RC489.A72E975 2005
  615.8′5156—dc22

                                                            2004019048

About the Editor

Cathy A. Malchiodi, ATR, LPCC, CPAT, is a licensed clinical mental health counselor, art therapist, and expressive arts therapist, and is also a faculty member at the National Institute for Trauma and Loss in Children. She has more than 20 years of clinical experience in working with people of all ages and has worked as an art therapist with survivors of traumatic experiences, including domestic violence, physical and sexual abuse, disaster, and serious or life-threatening illnesses. Ms. Malchiodi is a frequent presenter on art and health care throughout the United States, Canada, Asia, and Europe, and has given more than 200 invited presentations. She is the only person to have received all three of the American Art Therapy Association's highest honors: Distinguished Service Award (1991), Clinician Award (2000), and Honorary Life Member Award (2002). The author or editor of numerous books, including *The Art Therapy Sourcebook, Understanding Children's Drawings,* and the *Handbook of Art Therapy,* she has also published over 70 peer-reviewed papers on the use of art therapy and arts medicine with trauma survivors, survivors of child physical and sexual abuse, people with psychiatric disorders, and those with physical illness.

Contributors

Emily DeFrance, PhD, RPT-S, is Associate Professor in the Counseling Program at Sam Houston State University in Huntsville, Texas. She has also been a psychologist in private practice in Houston, Texas, for over 25 years. Dr. DeFrance has used play therapy with children of all ages, from a predominantly psychodynamic background, informed by humanistic theory. She also teaches two courses in play therapy and supervises play therapy interns through the university as well as in her private practice. She has been a presenter at the national level, and has been active in the Texas Association for Play Therapy as a member of the board of directors and in the Association for Play Therapy.

Karen Estrella, ATR-BC, MT-BC, LMHC, has been teaching expressive therapies at Lesley University in Cambridge, Massachusetts, since 1990. Ms. Estrella has over 20 years of experience practicing expressive therapies and mental health counseling, primarily in community-based mental health programs with a variety of clinical populations. She is also pursuing a PhD in clinical psychology at the Fielding Graduate Institute, where she integrates more traditional approaches to psychotherapy with expressive therapy and intermodal techniques. She is writing her dissertation on issues of social class identity and the psychotherapy supervisor, and has a particular interest in multicultural issues in therapy. In addition to teaching, she has a private practice in which she does counseling and psychotherapy, expressive arts therapy, and supervision.

Michele Forinash, DA, MT-BC, LMHC, is Associate Professor and coordinator of the music therapy specialization in the Division of Expressive Therapies at Lesley University in Cambridge, Massachusetts. Currently president of the American Music Therapy Association, Dr. Forinash is the editor of *Music Therapy Supervision* and coeditor of *Educators, Therapists, and Artists on Reflective Practice.* She has also published several articles and chapters on qualitative research in music therapy and is the North American editor for the online international music therapy journal *Voices: A World Forum for Music Therapy (www.voices.no).*

Kenneth Gorelick, MD, RPT, a psychiatrist in private practice and Clinical Professor of Psychiatry at George Washington University School of Medicine, has had experience as a clinician, a teacher, and an activist. He trained under Arleen Hynes at St. Elizabeths Hospital, where he worked with patients coping with schizophrenia and affective illnesses. Dr. Gorelick also served two terms as president of the National Association for Poetry Therapy (NAPT), was founding copresident of the NAPT Foundation, and served many years on the board of the National Federation for Biblio/PoetryTherapy. He has given workshops nationally and internationally in Russia, Turkey, and Italy.

Linda E. Homeyer, PhD, LPC, NCC, RPT-S, Associate Professor in the Professional Counseling Program at Texas State University–San Marcos, developed the play therapy training program at Texas State, including the first play therapy course available by distance learning. She is a frequent presenter at professional conferences and training throughout the United States and internationally. Dr. Homeyer is currently on the Association for Play Therapy's board of directors. She is coauthor of *Play Therapy with Children's Problems, The World of Play Therapy Literature,* as well as various chapters and journal articles, and coeditor (with Daniel S. Sweeney) of *The Handbook of Group Play Therapy.* She maintains a private practice in San Marcos, Texas.

Robert J. Landy, PhD, RDT/BCT, is Professor of Educational Theatre and the founder and director of the Drama Therapy Program at New York University, where he was a recipient of the Distinguished Teaching Medal. He has published numerous scholarly articles. His books include *Handbook of Educational Drama and Theatre; Drama Therapy: Concepts, Theories and Practices; Persona and Performance: The Meaning of Role in Drama, Therapy, and Everyday Life; Essays in Drama Therapy: The Double Life; New Essays in Drama Therapy: Unfinished Business;* and *How We See God and Why It Matters.* Dr. Landy is also a theatre artist whose musical play *God Lives in Glass* was recently produced at the Provincetown Playhouse in New York City.

Susan T. Loman, MA, ADTR, NCC, is the director of the Dance/Movement Therapy Program and associate chairperson, Department of Applied Psychology, Antioch New England Graduate School. She served as the chair of the education committee for the American Dance Therapy Association and is on the editorial board of *The Arts in Psychotherapy.* Ms. Loman directed the Creative Art Therapy Department at Billings Hospital's psychiatric unit; worked with infants, toddlers, and parents at the Center for Parents and Children; and worked with adults at Trenton Psychiatric Hospital. A Kestenberg Movement Profile (KMP) analyst, she worked closely with Judith Kestenberg for 8 years, chaired four conferences on the KMP, and has written numerous articles and coedited three books, including *The Meaning of Movement: Developmental and Clinical Perspectives of the Kestenberg Movement Profile.* She currently teaches the KMP system at Antioch New England Graduate School and taught the system at the Laban/Bartenieff Institute for Movement Studies in New York City for 14 years. She has lectured and conducted KMP workshops in Germany, England, Italy, Argentina, and the Netherlands, as well as throughout the United States.

Cathy A. Malchiodi (see "About the Editor").

Daniel S. Sweeney, PhD, LPC, LMFT, RPT-S, Associate Professor and Clinical Director in the Graduate Department of Counseling at George Fox University (GFU) in Portland, Oregon, is the director of the Northwest Center for Play Therapy Studies at GFU. He also has a private practice and has extensive experience in working with children, couples, and families. Dr. Sweeney has presented at many national and international conferences on the topics of play, filial, and sandtray therapy. He has numerous publications on child and family counseling, and is an author or coauthor of several books, including *Play Therapy Interventions with Children's Problems, Counseling Children through the World of Play,* and *Sandtray Therapy: A Practical Manual,* and coeditor (with Linda E. Homeyer) of *The Handbook of Group Play Therapy.* His books have been translated into Russian, French, and Mandarin.

Foreword

As a long-standing advocate for collaboration among all of the arts in therapy, it is reassuring to see Cathy Malchiodi, art therapy's preeminent editor and one of its most distinguished authors, committing herself to this vision and bringing it to a larger community of therapists. In compiling *Expressive Therapies,* Malchiodi has stepped across the lines of specialization and reached out to leading authors in sister disciplines to affirm the creative space that unites every form of expressive therapy.

All of the arts therapies, and the practices of play therapy and sandplay therapy that are also presented in this book, share features that distinguish them from what has been called "the talking cure"—a primary commitment to expressive action that engages emotions in a direct and physical way; an ability to generate creative energy as a healing force for mind, body, and spirit; and a belief that the creative imagination can find its way through our most perplexing and complex problems and conflicts. Each chapter provides a comprehensive description of the particular modality, including different theoretical and clinical approaches, methods of assessment, and vignettes of case experiences. This consistent format and the straightforward descriptions provided by each author result in a clearly organized handbook that will inform the work of experienced therapists while also offering an overview of the field for students and beginning practitioners.

The rise of the arts in therapy during the 1960s and 1970s was fueled by the values of expressionism in the arts, a more egalitarian approach to seeing the aesthetic significance of every person's expression, the desire of artists to use creative expression to serve others and society, the recognition that spoken language has many limits when it comes to communicating the total range of human emotions and experience, and the psychological realization that diverse forms of symbolic expression fulfill basic human needs. From the first days of expressive therapies practice, leading psychiatrists approached the different modalities with a sense of their ability to significantly accelerate and deepen the psychotherapeutic process, engaging people "more directly and more immediately than do any of the more traditional verbal therapies" (Zwerling, 1979, p. 843).

I first encountered the term "expressive therapy" when I was working as an art therapist in a Massachusetts state mental hospital in the early 1970s. The commissioner of mental health used the term "expressive therapy" to designate the use of all of the arts in therapy. There was an attempt to build bridges among the modalities and to create a strong new professional area that could participate as a peer with the older and larger disciplines of psychiatry, psychology, and social work. I embraced the opportunity to work with the Department of Mental Health in furthering innovative multidisciplinary training programs and founded the Expressive Therapies Graduate Program at Lesley University in 1974. Our model has been resilient and has spawned a number of similar training programs in Europe, Israel, Canada, and the United States. Together with colleagues in hundreds of college and university training programs, we have discovered that the use of the arts in healing has deep and lasting roots in human experience. Professionals in all parts of the world engage the arts to revitalize their professional practice, expand and enrich the expression of the people they serve, and bring creative energy and imagination to the organizations in which they work.

The original expressive therapists were inspired by visions of what the arts and the creative spirit can bring to the mental health field. The work was discovered independently by people in many different settings. This has resulted in a variety of practices and forms of professional organization, ranging from associations committed to single art modalities in mental health to others focused on integrating the arts. There are also new groups working to bring the arts to every sector of health care. All of these practices and many more belong together in a community that supports all attempts to promote the healing powers of art (McNiff, in press). There are therapists who claim expressive therapies as their primary professional identification and others in fields such as medicine, psychology, counseling, social work, nursing, education, and religious ministries who integrate expressive therapy methods into their practice. My greatest source of inspiration is how people in every region of the world, from children to the elderly, when confronted with life crises, serious illnesses, and tragedies, turn to creative expression as a way of engaging and transforming difficulties that cannot be healed in any other way.

This broad spectrum of practices and opportunities is a sign of the great appeal and the sustained relevance of the expressive therapies. I have always advocated that those of us who have committed our lives to the work need to avoid identification with values of narrow technical specialization that will only reinforce the adjunctive and often marginal status that the expressive therapies sometimes experienced when they began to grow in both North America and Europe. We need to reach out to every professional interested in becoming involved with expressive therapy methods. Since the scattering of the expressive therapies into disconnected groups can be viewed as a threat to their future vitality, the publication of this book and the collaboration displayed by its authors is a major contribution to the creation of a closer community of practice.

Over the past three decades expressive therapists throughout the world have secured a lasting place for their work through their clinical contributions, numerous publications, creation of training programs awarding advanced degrees, and the great imagination they have brought to expanding the place of art in healing to all sectors of society. The practice of expressive therapies that first took place in mental hospitals and clinics has now expanded to schools, hospices, community centers, disaster relief programs, churches, prisons, courts, cultural institutions, the workplace, and every conceivable setting committed to responding to the creative needs of people. These pioneering efforts have established a basis for an even greater growth of the work in the future. It is my hope that this book will inspire and guide a new generation of readers discovering how the expressive therapies can renew their professional and personal lives.

As we build a community of therapists committed to varied forms of expression in therapy, we can find inspiration in our shamanic forebears in every region of the world who used the arts, ritual, and the varied forms of symbolic expression to heal the soul. World history suggests that our methods of healing have always existed as a defining characteristic of human experience. Thus it is ironic how the expressive therapies, for so long struggling with the image of existing on the "fringes" of psychotherapy, are actually at the very core of the process and always have been.

At the beginning of the 20th century C. G. Jung anticipated everything we do today in the expressive therapies. In his practice of active imagination Jung understood how the hands working with clay, the body interpreting a dream through movement, or all of a person's expressive faculties dramatically enacting a conflict can offer insights and solutions that cannot be accessed through more linear verbal discussions. Even more in keeping with the core dynamics of the art experience, Jung experienced how the process of creation, without reliance on verbal explanation, heals by generating life-enhancing energies that revitalize the soul.

Where Freud used images as data for rational analysis, Jung approached the process of imagining and creating images as the "primary process" of his therapeutic and psychological inquiries—a very big difference indeed and one that secures Jung's place as the primary forerunner of expressive therapy within the modern psychological and mental health professions.

I hope that we can use Jung as an example of how a person, in this case a psychiatrist, who was not trained professionally in the arts, nevertheless used them in therapy with great effectiveness, intelligence, and creativity. Jung's practice of active imagination grew from his commitment to the different modes of expression, his passion for symbolic expression, and his complete personal immersion in the practices that he brought to his patients. By following Jung's example we both further the quality of creative expression in therapy and make it possible to expand our community of participants to other therapeutic disciplines.

I encourage readers of this book to imagine themselves as Jung; as deeply curious and interested in how all modes of creative expression can help people; as open to experimenting with new methods of expression in both your personal life and in your work with others; as willing to study these modes of expression, their history, and their symbolic qualities in an intelligent and comprehensive way; and as eager to learn from people with skills and interests and cultural backgrounds that are different from your own. I believe that the way Jung approached the practice of active imagination is a perfect model for reading and studying the chapters of this book and then applying them to our work with others.

Expression happens in therapy in so many ways. *Expressive Therapies* celebrates these varieties, from the exclusive use of one expressive modality to the discipline of integrating all of the arts that is so close to my heart. Each method offers a lifelong focus for a therapist's practice and skill enhancement. Within the community of expressive therapies there is room for all of these ways and many more. What matters is the realization that all creative modes of expression in therapy belong together and that they will renew your personal practice of therapy and therapy itself.

SHAUN MCNIFF, PHD
University Professor,
Lesley University,
Cambridge, Massachusetts

REFERENCES

McNiff, S. (in press). *Art heals: How creativity cures the soul.* Boston: Shambhala.

Zwerling, I. (1979). The creative arts therapies as "real therapies." *Hospital and Community Psychiatry, 30*(12), 841–844.

Preface

Effective therapists understand both their clients' styles of communication as well as how to bring out the best in their clients within the helping relationship. For more than 20 years as an art therapist and clinical mental health counselor, I have used the arts as a way of helping individuals gain new perspectives and become active participants in their own therapy. Whether with a grieving child, a family in distress, or an adult struggling with an emotional disorder, I continually have been impressed with the power of art and play to help people experience their world in new ways, communicate thoughts and feelings, induce positive change, and enhance health and well-being.

During the past 100 years, numerous individuals in the fields of psychology, psychiatry, counseling, creative arts therapies, and others have come to recognize the potential of art, music, movement, writing, drama, and other activities in therapy. "Expressive therapies" is one term often used to define this therapeutic use of the arts and play with children, adolescents, adults, families, and groups. Like verbal therapies, expressive therapies seek to facilitate change, communication, problem solving, and interpersonal skills, and to increase and enhance health and well-being in individuals of all ages. However, in contrast to strictly verbal therapies, these methods involve the purposeful, active participation of the individual and are often complemented by verbal interventions. As a result, these approaches encourage clients to engage in a process of self-expression with the objective of communicating feelings, thoughts, experiences, and perceptions in ways not always accomplished with words alone.

Expressive therapies have been applied to a wide range of client populations, including, but not limited to, those with psychiatric disorders, cognitive disabilities, trauma and loss, addictions, relationship problems, and developmental disorders. While creative arts therapists, expressive therapists, and play therapists make these therapies a central part of their work, helping professionals can easily adapt these approaches to their work with individuals, families, and groups. Counselors, psychologists, social workers, and marriage and family therapists also can apply the principles and practice described in this book and enhance their abilities to integrate a variety of creative methods in treatment.

Expressive Therapies provides a needed overview of the theory and practice of this rapidly increasing field and brings together experts in the fields of art therapy, music therapy, dance/movement therapy, drama therapy and psychodrama, poetry therapy, play therapy, and sandtray therapy, who delineate major approaches and demonstrate techniques with children, adolescents, and adults. In order to provide continuity, each chapter includes information on the major theoretical approaches of each modality, methods used in assessment and evaluation, and clinical applications with actual client populations. Professionals who are new to the field of expressive therapies will find pragmatic descriptions and case examples that will help them to apply these principles in their own work. Creative arts therapists, counselors, psychologists, and other mental health professionals who have advanced knowledge of expressive therapies will be treated to concise information on practice, theory, clinical applications, and field-tested methods from leading authors in the field.

Gladding and Newsome (2003) note that effective counseling "employs an artistic quality that enables individuals to express themselves in a creative and unique manner" (p. 251). The theories and techniques described in this volume offer therapists the opportunity to introduce imagination, play, energy, and creativity into the therapeutic process and enhance helping professionals' skills in guiding clients to express themselves in "creative and unique" ways. Expressive therapies offer unique ways to enhance communication as well as fresh directions for therapeutic work for both the client and therapist. It is my hope that readers of *Expressive Therapies* will be inspired by the extensive range of ideas, examples, and possibilities in the pages that follow and will deepen their own understanding of the value of expressive therapies as modalities for change and growth in their clients.

CATHY A. MALCHIODI

REFERENCE

Gladding, S., & Newsome, D. (2003). Art in counseling. In C. Malchiodi (Ed.), *Handbook of art therapy* (pp. 243–253). New York: Guilford Press.

Acknowledgments

It is with great respect that I take this opportunity to acknowledge several individuals in the field of expressive therapies who have helped to make this volume possible. While there are numerous experts who have formed the theoretical and methodological basis for the field, there are four individuals whose work has personally inspired me to initiate this book and to continue to make expressive therapies a central part of my work.

First, I want to thank Paolo Knill, Professor Emeritus, Lesley University Expressive Therapies Program, who supported my early work as an art therapist, expressive therapist, and author. Paolo's groundbreaking international work as a therapist, facilitator, and educator continues to influence the field of expressive therapies in the United States, Canada, and Europe, and his vision for the interrelated dimensions of the arts and therapy shaped the foundations of this book.

I also acknowledge Shaun McNiff, University Professor and founder of the Expressive Therapies Program at Lesley University, whose lasting commitment to the importance of imagination and self-expression as a form of "medicine" has served as an inspiration to the creation of this text. There is no one more worthy of writing the foreword of this book than Shaun, and I value his cogent historical perspective as well as encouragement of my work as an author and editor.

I next thank Susan Spaniol, Associate Professor and Director of the Art Therapy Specialization at Lesley University, for her unwavering support of my work and her warmth and wisdom as a friend and colleague.

Susan's seminal work in the area of arts and mental health has guided my thinking and enhanced the fields of both expressive therapies and mental health counseling.

I acknowledge as well Samuel T. Gladding, Provost and Professor, Wake Forest University, and President, American Counseling Association, for his visionary thinking on the importance of creativity in counseling and psychotherapy, his influential books and articles, and his recognition of the creative arts therapies as central to treatment and intervention.

In addition, I thank the authors—Michele Forinash, Susan T. Loman, Robert J. Landy, Kenneth Gorelick, Linda E. Homeyer, Emily DeFrance, Daniel S. Sweeney, and Karen Estrella—for graciously agreeing to write chapters for this text. These experts, each well known in his or her respective field, have provided both articulate and passionate summaries that illustrate the scope and potential of expressive therapies as agents of profound therapeutic change.

Finally, bringing together a book of this nature is never a solitary operation. I extend special thanks to the wonderful staff at The Guilford Press, especially Rochelle Serwator and Anna Nelson, for facilitating yet another pleasurable editorial experience and production process.

Contents

❧ 1

Expressive Therapies

History, Theory, and Practice

CATHY A. MALCHIODI

In his seminal work *The Arts and Psychotherapy*, McNiff (1981) observes that expressive therapies are those that introduce action to psychotherapy and that "action within therapy and life is rarely limited to a specific mode of expression" (p. viii). While talk is still the traditional method of exchange in therapy and counseling, practitioners of expressive therapies know that people also have different expressive styles—one individual may be more visual, another more tactile, and so forth. When therapists are able to include these various expressive capacities in their work with clients, they can more fully enhance each person's abilities to communicate effectively and authentically.

This chapter introduces readers to the history and philosophy of expressive therapies and their applications in treatment. While there are approximately 30,000 individuals throughout the United States formally trained at the graduate level in one or more of the expressive therapies, these modalities have also been embraced by practitioners in the fields of psychology, psychiatry, social work, counseling, and medicine over the last decade. Activities such as drawing, drumming, creative movement, and play permit individuals of all ages to express their thoughts and feelings in a manner that is different than strictly verbal means and have unique properties as interventions. Indeed, with the advent of brief

1

forms of treatment, many therapists find that the expressive therapies help individuals to quickly communicate relevant issues in ways that talk therapy cannot do. For this reason and others, psychologists, counselors, and other health care professionals are turning to expressive modalities in their work with individuals of all ages.

DEFINING EXPRESSIVE THERAPIES

The expressive therapies are defined in this text as the use of art, music, dance/movement, drama, poetry/creative writing, play, and sandtray within the context of psychotherapy, counseling, rehabilitation, or health care. Several of the expressive therapies are also considered "creative arts therapies"—specifically, art, music, dance/movement, drama, and poetry/creative writing according to the National Coalition of Creative Arts Therapies Associations (2004a; hereafter abbreviated as NCCATA). Additionally, expressive therapies are sometimes referred to as "integrative approaches" when purposively used in combination in treatment.

While expressive therapies can be considered a unique domain of psychotherapy and counseling, within this domain exists a set of individual approaches, defined as follows:

- *Art therapy* uses art media, images, and the creative process, and respects patient/client responses to the created products as reflections of development, abilities, personality, interests, concerns, and conflicts. It is a therapeutic means of reconciling emotional conflicts, fostering self-awareness, developing social skills, managing behavior, solving problems, reducing anxiety, aiding reality orientation, and increasing self-esteem (American Art Therapy Association, 2004).
- *Music therapy* uses music to effect positive changes in the psychological, physical, cognitive, or social functioning of individuals with health or educational problems (American Music Therapy Association, 2004).
- *Drama therapy* is the systematic and intentional use of drama/theatre processes, products, and associations to achieve the therapeutic goals of symptom relief, emotional and physical integration, and personal growth. It is an active approach that helps the client tell his or her story to solve a problem, achieve a catharsis, extend the depth and breadth of inner experience, understand the meaning of images, and

strengthen the ability to observe personal roles while increasing flexibility between roles (National Drama Therapy Association, 2004).

• *Dance/movement therapy* is based on the assumption that body and mind are interrelated and is defined as the psychotherapeutic use of movement as a process that furthers the emotional, cognitive, and physical integration of the individual. Dance/movement therapy effects changes in feelings, cognition, physical functioning, and behavior (NCCATA, 2004b).

• *Poetry therapy and bibliotherapy* are terms used synonymously to describe the intentional use of poetry and other forms of literature for healing and personal growth (NCCATA, 2004c).

• *Play therapy* is the systematic use of a theoretical model to establish an interpersonal process wherein trained play therapists use the therapeutic powers of play to help clients prevent or resolve psychosocial difficulties and achieve optimal growth and development (Boyd-Webb, 1999; Landreth, 1991).

• *Sandplay therapy* is a creative form of psychotherapy that uses a sandbox and a large collection of miniatures to enable a client to explore the deeper layers of the psyche in a totally new format. By constructing a series of "sand pictures," a client is helped to illustrate and integrate his or her psychological condition.

• *Integrated arts approach or intermodal (also known as multimodal) therapy* involves two or more expressive therapies to foster awareness, encourage emotional growth, and enhance relationships with others. Intermodal therapy distinguishes itself from its closely allied disciplines of art therapy, music therapy, dance/movement therapy, and drama therapy by being grounded in the interrelatedness of the arts. It is based on a variety of orientations, including arts as therapy, art psychotherapy, and the use of arts for traditional healing (Knill, Barba, & Fuchs, 1995).

Knill et al. (1995) observe that while all of the expressive therapies involve action, each also has inherent differences. For example, visual expression is conducive to more private, isolated work and may lend itself to enhancing the process of individuation; music often taps feeling and may lend itself to socialization when people collaborate in song or in simultaneously playing instruments; and dance/movement offer opportunities to interact and form relationships. In other words, each form of expressive therapy has its unique properties and roles in therapeutic work depending on its application, practitioner, client, setting, and objectives.

Therapists who are unfamiliar with expressive therapies often wonder if these modalities have been used as a form of assessment. Some practitioners of expressive therapies believe that using art, music, movement, or other modalities for evaluation is not practical due to a lack of substantive research data, and, that in some circumstances, such use may even be counterproductive. Despite this stance, formal assessments have been developed in art therapy, music therapy, and other expressive therapies for the purpose of adding to other available psychiatric, behavioral, and developmental assessments. Feder and Feder (1998) identify several basic ways in which the expressive therapies have been used in assessment: (1) assessment of abilities and preferences including formal and informal inventories and observations of individuals' skills and interests; (2) assessment of life experiences and capacities; and (3) assessment of psychological, psychosocial, and/or cognitive aspects. Many of these assessments, described throughout subsequent chapters of this book, may be used in combination with other evaluation methods in the related fields of psychology and counseling.

Finally, expressive therapies, such as art, music, and dance/movement, have been sometimes incorrectly labeled as "nonverbal" therapies. They are, in fact, both nonverbal and verbal because verbal communication of thoughts and feelings is a central part of therapy in most situations. However, for a child who has limited language, an elderly person who has lost the ability to talk because of a stroke or dementia, or a trauma victim who may be unable to put ideas into speech, expression through art, music, movement, or play can be ways to convey oneself without words and may be the primary form of communication in therapy.

A BRIEF HISTORY OF EXPRESSIVE THERAPIES

McNiff (1981, 1992) proposes that the arts have consistently been part of life as well as healing throughout the history of humankind. Today, expressive therapies have an increasingly recognized role in mental health, rehabilitation, and medicine. However, as McNiff observes, these therapies have been used since ancient times as preventative and reparative forms of treatment. There are numerous references within medicine, anthropology, and the arts to the earliest healing applications of expressive modalities. For example, the Egyptians are reported to have encouraged people with mental illness to engage in artistic activity (Fleshman & Fryrear, 1981); the Greeks used drama and music for its reparative properties (Gladding, 1992); and the story of King Saul in the Bible describes music's calming attributes. Later, in Europe during the Renaissance, English physician and writer Robert Burton theorized that imagination played a role in health and well-being, while Italian philosopher de Feltre proposed that dance and play were central to children's healthy growth and development (Coughlin, 1990).

The idea of using the arts as an adjunct to medical treatment emerged in the period from the late 1800s to the 1900s alongside the advent of psychiatry. During this time the movement to provide more human treatment of people with mental illness began and "moral therapy" included patient involvement with the arts (Fleshman & Fryrear, 1981). While late-19th-century programs were transitory, the ideas behind them resurfaced in the early 1900s. For example, documented uses of music as therapy can be found following World War I when "miracle cures" were reported, resulting from reaching patients through music when they responded to nothing else. Joseph Moreno (1923), the founder of psychodrama, proposed the use of enactment as a way to restore mental health. He also described the use of positive creative imagery, role reversal, and "monodrama" (in which a participant enacts all parts of the self). At the same time, Florence Goodenough (1926) studied children's drawings as measures of cognitive development, and others, like Hans Prinzhorn, became interested in the art of patients with severe mental illnesses (Vick, 2003). Finally, the fields of sandplay, sandtray therapy, and the foundations of play therapy were present in Margaret Lowenfeld's "World Technique" in the 1920s (Lowenfeld, 1969). Lowenfeld began her training as a pediatrician and subsequently began to make observations about children's play, developing a method of using toys to understand psychosocial aspects of child clients.

The creative arts therapies became more widely known during the 1930s and 1940s when psychotherapists and artists began to realize that self-expression through nonverbal methods such as painting, music making, or movement might be helpful for people with severe mental illness. Because there were many patients for whom the "talking cure" was impractical, the arts therapies gradually began to find a place in treatment. Major psychiatric hospitals such as the Menninger Clinic in Kansas and St. Elizabeths in Washington, DC, incorporated the arts within treatment, both as activity therapies and as modalities with psychotherapeutic benefits.

Professional associations for practitioners of art, music, and other expressive therapies were established and university programs training practitioners in these modalities rapidly developed. Over the last several decades, play therapy and sandplay therapy have also become part of expressive therapies practice and have developed specific theoretical foundations, methodologies, training, and professional associations. More recently, expressive therapies have been incorporated into a variety of mental health, rehabilitative, and medical settings as both primary and adjunctive forms of treatment. For example, music and imagery therapies are now used routinely with hospitalized patients for pain reduction, relaxation, and childbirth; art and play are proving to be essential in trauma debriefing, resolution, and recovery with children (Malchiodi, 2001); and writing is prescribed to ameliorate symptoms of illnesses such as asthma and arthritis as well as to decrease posttraumatic stress in individuals who have experienced crisis or loss (Pennebaker, 1997).

EDUCATION, COMPETENCY, AND STANDARDS OF PRACTICE

Many practitioners who incorporate the expressive therapies into the practice of psychotherapy have studied these modalities through graduate-level training and may hold a credential in one or more of the media they use. These practitioners are distinguished by credentials in art therapy, music therapy, play therapy, and so forth, either in the form of a master's or doctoral degree, or through registration, certification, or licensure in a specific creative art therapy or expressive therapy (see the Appendix for a list of professional associations). Those therapists whose training has included multiple modalities are often referred to as "expressive arts therapists" or "expressive therapists." Knill et al. (1995) propose that those who take an integrated approach (see Chapter 9) do not need to master all forms of expressive therapy. They observe that it is more important to have a focus on the artistic tradition that all expressive therapies have in common: human imagination. This is the same tradition that healers throughout history used who did not divide their work into specializations of drumming, art making, or ritual; rather, they used multimodal aspects in their work. Knill et al. conclude that using more than one modality in therapy is more efficacious and helps therapists to avoid the trap that Maslow is quoted as saying "If the only tool you have is a hammer, every problem starts to look like a nail."

In terms of training, a discussion within expressive therapies continues about the importance and role of in-depth training in an art form through studio work in order to practice creative interventions. Some believe that in order for a therapist to be effective, he or she must have had significant experiences in art, music, dance, drama, poetry, play, or sandtray in order to competently and ethically use these modalities in therapy. With regard to art therapy, Agell (1982) notes that "a flirtation with materials is not enough. Only a love affair with materials can lead to a wedding of felt experience and formed expression" (p. 37). While many therapists are familiar with several expressive therapies, generally most tend to specialize in one or two that they are trained in and that meet the needs and situation of their clients. Others, such as Gladding (1992) and Carson and Becker (2004), see expressive therapies as part of larger realm of "creativity in counseling." They propose that creativity in counseling involves being able to flexibly respond to clients with a variety of techniques and to encourage creativity within therapy. Carson and Becker (2004) note that there is a need for "counselors to be continually cultivating and nurturing their own creativity" (p. 114), although they do not offer any specific ideas or recommendations on how counselors and other mental health professionals can achieve this depth of knowledge.

Depending on the practitioner and the setting, expressive therapies may be used as a primary form of therapy, requiring the therapist to have a deeper understanding of how various modalities can be applied in response to a wide range of disorders. Often, expressive therapies are integrated within a psychotherapy or counseling framework. For example, Gladding and Newsome (2003) highlight the integration of visual art activities into counseling treatment plans with adults and emphasize that a quick client drawing or collage can move a client forward when talk therapy is resisted or ineffective. Also, many expressive therapy techniques have been used to complement a wide range of psychotherapy and counseling theories, including psychoanalytic, object relations, cognitive-behavioral, humanistic, transpersonal, and others (Malchiodi, 1998, 2003).

Finally, when using expressive therapies to complement verbal therapy, practitioners should be aware of the current standards of practice in the particular modality they are using. The American Art Therapy Association (AATA), the American Music Therapy Association (AMTA), the American Dance Therapy Association (ADTA), the National Drama Therapy Association (NADT), the National Poetry Therapy Association (NAPT), and the Association of Play Therapy (APT) all provide helpful guidelines about the application and practice of expressive modalities with clients in mental health, rehabilitation, special education, and health care settings. The NCCATA also offers information on standards of practice, training opportunities, and other subjects useful for practitioners. Additionally, each association has ethical standards that therapists who plan to use expressive therapies as a form of treatment or assessment should consult before integrating art, music, movement, play, or other methods into their work.

EXPRESSIVE THERAPIES' ROLE
IN TREATMENT AND INTERVENTION

In general, like counseling or psychotherapy, an expressive therapies session may open with a discussion of the individual's, family's, or group's goals, concerns, or current problems. In contrast to therapists who explore these issues through talking, expressive therapists encourage individuals to use an expressive form of communication as a means for further exploration. For example, clients may be asked to draw an image of an idea, enact a situation or engage in a dramatic dialogue, manipulate a set of figures in a sandtray, write a short story or poem, play with toys or props, or use a musical instrument to express a feeling. Depending on the client, the therapist may also begin a session with a warm-up activity or exercise such as a quick scribble, stretches, simple movements, or humming a familiar tune. The opening activity may be used simply for relaxation, to introduce a modality into the session, or to help the therapist evaluate the individual's mood or current concerns. One or more expressive therapies may be used in a session—for example, while a drama therapy session may involve role play, it is also likely to involve movement or may start with some creative writing or a piece of poetry to stimulate or inspire the invention of a story. In subsequent chapters, applications and case examples of expressive therapies, including integrative approaches, are described in detail, illustrating their vast range of application as primary therapies and as complements to verbal therapy from a variety of theoretical models.

UNIQUE CHARACTERISTICS
OF EXPRESSIVE THERAPIES

Expressive therapies add a unique dimension to psychotherapy and counseling because they have several specific characteristics not always found in strictly verbal therapies, including, but not limited to, (1) self-expression, (2) active participation, (3) imagination, and (4) mind–body connections.

Self-Expression

All therapies, by their very nature and purpose, encourage individuals to engage in self-exploration. Expressive therapies encourage not only self-exploration, but also use self-expression through one or more modalities as a central part of the therapeutic process. Gladding (1992) notes that using the arts in counseling may actually speed up the process of self-exploration and that expressive modalities allow people to experience themselves differently. He adds that through these forms of self-expression, individuals are able to "exhibit and practice novel and adaptive behaviors" (p. 6).

Self-expression through a painting, movement, or poem can recapitulate past experiences and even be cathartic for some, but these are only two aspects of the role of self-expression in therapy. In fact, most therapists using expressive therapies in their work capitalize on the ability of art, music, play, and other forms to contain self-expression rather than to encourage cathartic communication of raw emotions or mere repetition of troubling memories. In essence, as therapist and client work together, self-expression is used as a container for feelings and perceptions that may deepen into greater self-understanding or may be transformed, resulting in emotional reparation, resolution of conflicts, and a sense of well-being.

Expressive therapists generally do not seek to interpret individuals' drawings, movement, poems, or play, but instead try to facilitate their clients' discovery of personal meaning and understanding. For that reason, self-expression in an expressive therapies session also generally involves verbal reflection in order to help individuals to make sense of their experiences, feelings, and perceptions. While words are generally used to tell personal stories, expressive therapies are used to tap the senses as a source of stories and memories. Because thoughts and feelings are not strictly verbal and are not limited to storage as verbal language in the brain, expressive modalities are particularly useful in helping people communicate aspects of memories and stories that may not be readily available through conversation. Memories in particular have been reported to emerge through touch, imagery, or carefully guided body movements (Rothschild, 2000). For some individuals, telling a story through one or more expressive modality is more easily tolerated than verbalization. Individuals can "experience" their story, allowing the practitioner to capitalize on clients' discoveries and use the activity to help them broaden their understanding.

Some therapists believe that the process of expressive therapy (the telling of a story through an expressive modality such as art, music, movement, etc.) offers as much therapeutic value as verbal reflection about the product or experience. Landreth (1991), a well-known play therapy pioneer, notes that this holds particularly true for young children who do not have the verbal capabilities necessary for reflection through language. Expression through a painting, play activity, imaginative role play, or movement may be a corrective experience, in and of itself, for some individuals.

In cases where self-expression is repetitive, rigid, or noncorrective, a therapist using expressive techniques will actively engage with clients in order to help therapy progress. Art and play therapist Eliana Gil (1998) notes that when a child who has been severely traumatized repeats a play or art activity without resolution or correction the therapist must introduce activities or directives to help the child transform the storyline into a more productive and satisfying experience. Other therapists encourage client dialogues that involve "talking to the painting" (McNiff, 1992) or use an expressive modality as a source of reflection and exploration. For example, a poem can be written about a drawing, a painting can be made about a movement, a short play can be enacted about a piece of music, and so forth. Throughout this book readers will find examples of how this is accomplished, using expressive therapies as the basis.

Active Participation

Expressive therapies are defined by psychology as "action therapies" (Weiner, 1999) because they are action-oriented methods through which clients explore issues and communicate their thoughts and feelings. Art and music making, dance and drama, creative writing, and all forms of play are participatory and require individuals to invest energy in them. For example, art making, even in its simplest sense, can involve arranging, touching, gluing, stapling, painting, forming, and many other tangible experiences. All expressive therapies focus on encouraging clients to become active participants in the therapeutic process. The experience of doing, making, and creating can actually energize individuals, redirect attention and focus, and alleviate emotional stress, allowing clients to fully concentrate on issues, goals, and behaviors. Finally, in addition to promoting active participation, expressive therapies are sensory in nature. Many or all of the senses are utilized in one way or another when a person engages in art making, music playing or listening, dancing or moving, enacting, or playing. These types of activities and experiences redirect awareness to visual, tactile, and auditory channels.

Imagination

Levine (1999) observes that "imagination is the central concept which informs the understanding of the use of arts and play in therapy" (p. 259). McNiff (1981, 1992) believes that imagination is the healing agent inherent to all forms of self-expression. While some favor the use of the word "creativity" in describing expressive therapies, it is actually the use of imagination that informs theory and practice. In contrast to imagination, creativity occurs when self-expression is fully formed and achieves a novel and aesthetic value. In an expressive therapies session clients may not always make drawings, music, movements, or poems that would be considered creative or fully formed, but in most cases imaginative thinking is used to generate self-expression, experimentation, and subsequent verbal reflection.

The role of imagination in expressive therapies practice is illustrated throughout this book, but there are several specific qualities that are central to art, music, dance, drama, creative writing, and play in therapy. These modalities are helpful in assisting individuals in moving beyond their preconceived beliefs through experimentation with new ways of communication and experiences that involve "pretend." The imaginative thinking needed to make a drawing, create a movement, or manipulate figures in a sandtray also offers the possibility for trying out inventive solutions and transformation. Clients who may be otherwise restricted in their ability to use imagination in problem solving often find expressive therapies particularly helpful. For example, a person who has been severely traumatized may feel emotionally constricted or may have obsessive thoughts or memories. The therapeutic use of art, play, or sandtray can augment the productive use of imagination, helping the individual discover and develop corrective solutions leading to change, resolution, and reparation.

Mind–Body Connections

The National Center for Complementary and Alternative Medicine (2004; hereafter abbreviated as NCCAM) has defined mind–body interventions as those that are designed to facilitate the mind's capacity to influence bodily functions and symptoms. Many of the expressive therapies are considered by NCCAM to be mind–body interventions because they are both forms of psychotherapy and therapies that capitalize on the use of the senses to effect change. The advances made in the field of neuroscience and neurodevelopment have also drawn attention to the potential of expressive therapies in regard to mind–body intervention, particularly in the areas of mood disorders, stress disorders, and physical illness. For example, art, drama, and play therapies show promise in the amelioration of posttraumatic stress and the expression of traumatic memories. Music, art, and dance/movement may be helpful in tapping the body's relaxation response, a calm and confident state of being associated with perceptions of health, wellness, and happiness (Benson, 1996). Writing has proven to be effective in emotional reparation and in reducing symptoms in some chronic illnesses (Pennebaker, 1997). Overall, expressive activities may stimulate the placebo effect through mimicking self-soothing experiences of childhood and inducing self-relaxation (Malchiodi, 2003; Tinnin, 1994).

Finally, research on early attachment and brain development is beginning to inform psychotherapy of the value of expressive therapies. Expressive therapies, particularly dance, art, and play therapies, may be useful in reestablishing and encouraging healthy attachments through sensory experiences, interactions, movement, and hands-on activities. These modalities may be helpful in repairing and reshaping attachment through experiential and sensory means and may tap early relational states before words are dominant, possibly allowing the brain to establish new, more productive patterns (Malchiodi, 2003; Riley, 2002).

LIMITATIONS OF EXPRESSIVE THERAPIES

Like any therapy, there are limitations to expressive therapy in treatment and intervention. While expressive therapies have been applied to all age groups, to most psychiatric and medical disorders, and to a variety of settings, there are clients who may not benefit from these modalities for various reasons. First, some individuals, often adults, may be hesitant to engage in an expressive modality in therapy because they believe they are not "creative" or cannot produce something that is "artistic." Therapists initiating expressive activities as interventions may encounter resistance to participation by clients who perceive themselves as unable to use imagination, who are anxious about self-expression, or who are resistant to active participation. Additionally, and ironically, those individuals with extensive experience in painting, music, or dance may not be able to let go of learned rules about self-expression and may be inhibited in their spontaneity in therapy when asked to express themselves in their particular medium.

For therapists who have not had extensive training in expressive therapies, there may be a tendency to want to interpret what their clients do in a given modality. This is particularly true of client-created drawings and other art expressions; practitioners may be tempted to project their own conclusions about content, sometimes missing their clients' intended meanings. Additionally, therapists without experience may use expressive modalities in a mechanical fashion and use activities and techniques routinely rather than thinking about what would be best for clients given their histories, presenting problems and potentials, and goals. Because expressive therapies can include directed activities, it is easy for some therapists to fall into the habit of simply choosing an expressive activity or directive from a book or workshop. As with any form of therapy, it is important to listen to and respect what the client is communicating and then create an intervention that is best suited to the individual's needs and objectives.

Finally, while research on the efficacy of expressive therapies is increasing dramatically, there is still much to be learned about how they work and how they should be applied in work with children, adults, families, and groups. Music therapy is possibly the most widely researched modality, largely because physiological and behavioral reactions to music and music therapy interventions can be quantified. Within the field of art therapy, art-based assessments have been more extensively studied and efficacy studies in the areas of trauma and emotional disorders are receiving more attention (Malchiodi, 2003). In brief, while there have been some qualitative studies in the expressive therapies, most of the literature discusses clinical observations, case examples, and applications. Because of the recognition by mental health professionals of the inherent value of expressive modalities in treatment, interest in research is increasing, particularly in the areas of trauma, mood disorders, Alzheimer's disease and other forms of dementia, and childhood disorders such as attention-deficit/hyperactivity disorder and autism.

CONCLUSION

Johnson (1985) observes that expressive therapists "have a powerful vision, and we have emerged for a reason" (p. 238). In the same vein, the expressive therapies as a force with psychology and counseling have emerged for a reason. A growing number of mental health professionals are recognizing why expressive therapies enhance work with clients in ways that strictly verbal therapies cannot. Additionally, there is a growing movement in mental health to utilize "creative methods" in therapy and medicine.

Creativity in therapy has the potential to impact clients in memorable ways that traditional interventions do not. When therapists choose to use expressive therapies, they give their clients the opportunity to become active participants in their own treatment and empower them to use imagination in productive and corrective ways. Whether through art, play, music, movement, enactment, or creative writing, expressive therapies stimulate the senses, thereby "sensitizing" individuals to untapped aspects of themselves (Gladding, 1991) and thus facilitating self-discovery, change, and reparation.

REFERENCES

Agell, G. (1982). The place of art in art therapy: Art therapy or arts therapy. *American Journal of Art Therapy, 21*, 15–18.
American Art Therapy Association. (2004). *About art therapy* [Online]. Available at *www.arttherapy.org*.
American Music Therapy Association. (2004). *Definition of music therapy* [Online]. Available at *www.musictherapy.org*.
Benson, H. (1996). *Timeless healing: The power and biology of belief*. New York: Scribner's.
Boyd-Webb, N. (Ed.). (1999). *Play therapy with children in crisis* (2nd ed.). New York: Guilford Press.
Carson, D., & Becker, K. (2004). When lightning strikes: Reexamining creativity in psychotherapy. *Journal of Counseling and Development, 82*(1), 111–115.
Coughlin, E. (1990). Renewed appreciation of connections between mind and body stimulate researchers to harness the healing power of the arts. *Chronicles of Higher Education, 36*, 9.
Feder, B., & Feder, E. (1998). *The art and science of evaluation in the arts therapies: How do you know what's working?* Springfield, IL: Thomas.
Fleshman, B., & Fryrear, J. (1981). *The arts in therapy*. Chicago: Nelson-Hall.
Gil, E. (1998). *Play therapy for severe psychological trauma* [Videotape]. New York: Guilford Press.
Gladding, S. (1992). *Counseling as an art: The creative arts in counseling*. Alexandria, VA: American Counseling Association.
Gladding, S. T., & Newsome, D. W. (2003). Art in counseling. In C. A. Malchiodi (Ed.), *Handbook of art therapy* (pp. 243–253). New York: Guilford Press.

Goodenough, F. (1926). *Measurement of intelligence by drawings.* New York: Harcourt, Brace, & World.

Johnson, D. R. (1985). Envisioning the link among the creative arts therapies. *Arts in Psychotherapy, 12*(4), 233–238.

Knill, P., Barba, H., & Fuchs, M. (1995). *Minstrels of the soul.* Toronto: Palmerston Press.

Landreth, G. (1991). *Play therapy: The art of relationship.* Muncie, IN: Accelerated Development.

Levine, E. (1999). On the play ground: Child psychotherapy and expressive arts therapy. In S. Levine & E. Levine (Eds.), *Foundations of expressive arts therapy: Theoretical and clinical perspectives* (pp. 257–273). London: Kingsley.

Lowenfeld, M. (1969). *The world technique.* London: Allen & Unwin.

Malchiodi, C. A. (1998). *The art therapy sourcebook.* New York: McGraw-Hill/ Contemporary Books.

Malchiodi, C. A. (2001). Using drawings as interventions with traumatized children. *Trauma and Loss: Research and Interventions, 1*(1), 21–27.

Malchiodi, C. A. (Ed.). (2003). *Handbook of art therapy.* New York: Guilford Press.

McNiff, S. (1981). *The arts and psychotherapy.* Springfield, IL: Thomas.

McNiff. S. (1992). *Art and medicine.* Boston: Shambhala.

Moreno, J. (1923). *Das Stegif Theater.* Berlin: Gustave Kiepenheur.

National Center for Complementary and Alternative Medicine. (2004). *Major domains of complementary and alternative medicine* [Online]. Available at *nccam.nih.gov/fcp/classify/.*

National Coalition of Creative Arts Therapies Associations. (2004a). *National Coalition of Creative Arts Therapies Associations* [Online]. Available at *www.nccata.org/.*

National Coalition of Creative Arts Therapies Associations. (2004b). *Dance/ movement therapy* [Online]. Available at *www.nccata.org/dance.html.*

National Coalition of Creative Arts Therapies Associations. (2004c). *Poetry therapy* [Online]. Available at *www.nccata.org/poetry.html.*

National Drama Therapy Association. (2004). *General questions about drama therapy* [Online]. Available at *www.nadt.org/.*

Pennebaker, J. W. (1997). *Opening up: The healing power of expressing emotions.* New York: Guilford Press.

Riley, S. (2001). *Group process made visible.* New York: Brunner-Routledge.

Rothschild, B. (2000). *The body remembers: The psychobiology of trauma and trauma treatment.* New York: Norton.

Tinnin, L. (1994). Transforming the placebo effect in art therapy. *American Journal of Art Therapy, 32*(3), 75–78.

Vick, R. M. (2003). A brief history of art therapy. In C. A. Malchiodi (Ed.), *Handbook of art therapy* (pp. 5–15). New York: Guilford Press.

Weiner, D. (1999). Beyond talk therapy: Using movement and expressive techniques in clinical practice. Washington, DC: American Psychological Association.

2

Art Therapy

CATHY A. MALCHIODI

Throughout the history of psychiatry and psychology, practitioners have had a natural attraction to the use of art expression in work with their clients. As early as 1912, German psychiatrists Emil Kraepelin and Karl Jaspers observed that drawings by patients could be used as aids in understanding psychopathology. The theories of Freud and Jung supported the idea that art expression and images have an important place in psychiatric evaluation and treatment. Freud posited the existence of an unconscious mind and an inner world of meaningful fantasies and dreams, while Jung believed in universal archetypes and symbols and explored his own psyche and that of his patients through art expression.

Despite the long-standing interest in art and mental health, art therapy as a definable method of practice has only existed since the mid-20th century. During the 1940s, British artist Adrian Hill observed the value of art making during his stay as a tuberculosis patient at a sanatorium. Hill believed that art making was a form of therapy and, by his own account, he was the first art therapist. Simultaneously, in the United States, Margaret Naumburg noted that art expression was a way to manifest unconscious imagery, an observation resonant with the predominant psychoanalytic viewpoint of the times. Naumburg is considered to be one of the earliest practitioners to delineate art therapy as a distinct form of psychotherapy, proposing that images produced by clients were a form of symbolic speech. Others, like child psychiatrist Donald Winnicott (1971), promoted the value of art as a transitional object and creative activity as a reflection of thoughts, feelings, fantasies, and conflicts. By the 1970s, art therapy had emerged as a field with specialized approaches to assessment and clinical practice.

While art therapy is now considered a profession with specialized education, credentials, and standards of practice, art expression is also widely utilized by counselors, social workers, psychologists, play therapists, and others as a form of intervention. For example, therapists who work with children invariably find that they must include experiential activities in order to engage young clients and to provide them with a developmentally meaningful form of expression. Counselors often use drawing and collage making in their work with a variety of child and adult populations, tailoring activities to meet the specific needs of clients and the goals of treatment (Gladding & Newsome, 2003). As psychology becomes increasingly informed by discoveries in neuroscience, and particularly with how the brain stores memories and images, more clinicians are becoming interested in the application of sensory-based therapies such as art therapy in their work (Malchiodi, 2003).

DEFINITION AND SCOPE OF PRACTICE

If you ask art therapists to define art therapy, you generally receive many different responses. Some define art therapy as a method of treatment that is based on the use of art as a form of communication and self-expression. Others believe that art therapy is more complex than a simple replacement for verbalization. In this sense, the experience of creating images is believed to be inherently healing and to offer individuals a way to self-understanding, behavioral change, and emotional reparation.

Vick (2003) observes that art therapy is actually a hybrid discipline that draws from the fields of art and psychology. The integration of these two fields generated two general theories about how and why art therapy is useful as both a primary intervention and as an adjunctive modality. First, art expression is thought to be a form of visual language through which people can express thoughts and feelings that they cannot put into words. Second, it is a way to communicate experiences that are difficult to verbalize, such as physical or sexual abuse, trauma, grief, and other complex emotional experiences. While images may reveal aspects of the person who created them, an important part of the process of art therapy includes facilitating the individual's discovery of personal meaning for art expressions.

The American Art Therapy Association (1996) notes that art therapy is based on the belief that the "creative process of art making is healing and life-enhancing." In other words, art expression is helpful in overcoming emotional distress, resolving conflicts, achieving insights, reducing problematic behaviors, and increasing a sense of well-being. For example, making a painting of one's feelings may increase an individual's self-awareness; creating clay sculptures may be a form of relaxation and stress reduction for a person experiencing anxiety; assembling photo collages may be empowering for an adolescent with cancer or other serious illness; or relearning motor and perceptual skills through specific drawing tasks may be helpful to an older adult who has suffered a stroke. While art expression may be used as another form of language in therapy, the actual act of making art taps the universal human potential to be creative, a capacity that has been related to health and wellness (Malchiodi, 2002).

The definition and scope of art therapy have been influenced in part by the numerous mental health and medical settings in which art expression has been used as a form of intervention. Historically, art therapy has been used in psychiatric and day treatment facilities as part of overall services to people with mental illness. However, as health care has evolved, art therapy has been used with a growing variety of patient populations, including those suffering from substance abuse, trauma and loss, domestic violence, physical and sexual abuse, eating disorders, behavioral disorders, and most forms of mental illness. It has also been used as an intervention with individuals with attention-deficit/hyperactivity disorder (ADHD), autism, neurological problems, mental retardation, and other disorders. As preventative health programs emerge, art therapy has become increasingly prevalent in medical settings and has been integrated within both traditional and complementary forms of medical intervention (Councill, 2003; Malchiodi, 1998a, 1999). While most clinicians think of art expression as a form of play, and therefore most appropriate in work with children, art therapy is widely used with individual adults, couples, and families, and groups of all ages.

BENEFITS OF ART THERAPY

While there are still relatively few outcome studies that prove the effectiveness of art therapy with various patient populations, there are characteristics of art therapy that differentiate it from strictly verbal therapy and highlight its benefits as a form of treatment. First and foremost, while most therapy depends on words to convey meaning, art therapy provides the client with an opportunity to externalize his or her thoughts and feelings through visual images. Making an image, whether a drawing, a painting, or a sculpture, is an experience of visual thinking and can be an additional source of information for both client and therapist.

Art making, whether in the form of a simple pencil drawing or a more elaborate painting or sculpture, is experiential in nature because it utilizes the senses: touch, sight, and to some extent sound and smell. Like music, movement, and other expressive arts therapies, art therapy involves physical action, kinesthetic qualities, and perceptual experiences. It is a hands-on activity that can include drawing, constructing, arranging, mixing, touching, painting, forming, and other tangible actions. Because it is a modality that involves the body, it adds another dimension to verbal therapy or it can be used as an intervention in and of itself, depending on the goals of treatment.

Art expression offers a tangible and lasting product that provides a valuable component to therapy. Art also functions as a transitional object in that it is a concrete record of therapy and a reminder of the client–therapist relationship between meetings. A drawing or painting can be looked at, referred to, and talked about immediately or in a later session. For some individuals, looking at a drawing with a therapist may be easier than making eye contact with one another. Talking about an image and its meaning may be less difficult than talking directly to the therapist about sensitive or complex issues.

Art expression has also been promoted as helpful in releasing emotions. In psychological terms, this is known as *catharsis*, the discharge of strong emotions for relief. Making a drawing or a painting and discussing one's images within the context of therapy can be cathartic in that it may well provide the release of painful or troubling feelings. Engaging in art expression, because it stimulates the release of feelings, may actually increase verbal communication, recall of details, and the comfort level between therapist and client (Gross & Haynes, 1998).

The creative process of art making can also alleviate stress by inducing the physiological response of relaxation or by altering mood. For this reason, in addition to its benefits as a form of psychotherapy, art therapy has been defined as a "mind–body" intervention by the National Institutes of Health and categorized as a form of complementary medicine. As neuroscience continues to provide insights concerning the complex relationship between physiology, emotions, and images, art therapy's effectiveness is becoming more clearly understood (Malchiodi, 2003).

THE ROLE OF ART MATERIALS IN ART THERAPY

Art materials are part of what differentiate art therapy from strictly verbal therapy as well as from other forms of expressive therapy. A variety of art materials are used in art therapy, ranging from simple pencil drawing to more technologically complex forms of visual expression such as photography (Weiser, 1993) and computer-assisted image making (Malchiodi, 2000). Materials with which to draw, paint, sculpt, and create a collage form the standard media used in most art therapy sessions because they are easy to use, transportable, and accommodate a variety of settings. To some extent, the prevalence of brief treatment has influenced how art therapy is used in clinical practice. Because individual and some group sessions may only be an hour in length, using simple materials is necessary to meet the restraints of time and settings which may be an office desktop, a bed tray, or other limited space.

Art therapists generally develop treatment plans for clients based in part on the affective qualities of art media, selecting materials that best complement the goals of intervention. The size and texture of paper, specific paint and brushes, or a certain type of clay may be selected by the therapist to facilitate self-expression, complement therapeutic goals, or address individual preferences. For example, in a session focusing on family-of-origin issues, the therapist might offer modeling clay to encourage an individual to create a figure of each family member. Clay, as opposed to drawing, offers the possibility for making three-dimensional objects that are moveable in relation to each other. In this case, the goal of the intervention may be to help the individual literally work with family dynamics through creating and moving the individual clay figures. In contrast, a therapist may choose 8½" × 11" paper and colored pencils or felt markers for a child who has problems with impulse control because these materials are more easily controlled by the child and are less messy and stimulating than paints or clay.

ART-BASED ASSESSMENT

Therapists often use drawings or other art-based assessments to evaluate and understand children, adolescents, and adults and to assist in developing treatment plans. Projective drawing assessments that emerged during the first half of the 20th century have been used in psychology, psychiatry, and art therapy, although there has been criticism about their reliability and validity (Lillienfield, Wood, & Grab, 2000; Wadeson, 2002). Popular projective techniques include the House–Tree–Person drawings (HTP; Buck, 1949), Draw-A-Person (DAP) or human figure drawings (Koppitz, 1968), and the Kinetic Family Drawing (KFD; Burns & Kaufman, 1972). Psychoanalytic theories and, to some extent, developmental theories have greatly influenced much of the literature on how to evaluate these drawings.

The field of art therapy has developed its own art-based assessments, partly in response to the lack of reliability and validity of traditional projective drawing tasks. Contemporary researchers have favored methods that underscore the expressive potential of materials and the structural qualities of drawings over specific symbolic characteristics or elements; the Formal Elements Arts Therapy Scale (FEATS; Gantt & Tabone, 2003) and the Diagnostic Drawing Series (DDS; Mills, 2003) are two examples of this approach to understanding drawings. Both use scales to evaluate structural elements, color, and compositional aspects of specific standardized drawing tasks.

Other researchers have studied the content of and the verbal associations with standardized drawing tasks. The Silver Drawing Test (SDT; Silver, 2003) is a good example of this approach and includes the use of a series of specific images referred to as "stimulus drawings" and the directive to choose two of these images to create a drawing. The individual is also asked to provide a title and a short story about the drawing. Silver's initial goal was to identify creative and cognitive abilities in children, adolescents, and adults. Later, she became interested in the identification of depression and aggressive behaviors in children and adolescents and developed a 5-point Likert scale to evaluate whether the drawing and a story about the image had positive, neutral, or negative associations.

The field of art therapy has also generated assessments that do not necessarily provide conclusive information, but do provide ways to evaluate how clients express themselves through art and help to plan for future treatment. For example, art therapist Edith Kramer developed an assessment with children in order to evaluate how children create in three media: drawing, painting, and clay sculpture (Kramer & Schehr, 1983). Observing how a child works with each of these materials generates information on how and what the child expresses through art, as well as his or her abilities and preferences for specific media. In using this type of assessment, the therapist might compare the themes and content of each art product; determine if the child creates a developmentally appropriate expression or regresses into play activity; and observe whether the child prefers one material over another or is more fluent in drawing, painting, or clay sculpture. This information can serve as a foundation for subsequent treatment plans involving art-making directives or choosing specific materials. For example, a child may not be particularly skilled in drawing, but may be more comfortable constructing objects in clay. The same child may be regressive in using paint, preferring to play with the materials rather than create a fully formed art expression.

Some art therapists have argued that using art expression for assessment or diagnosis is nonproductive and generally nonconclusive, while others have observed that drawings and other art products offer important assessment data under certain circumstances (Williams, Agell, Gantt, & Goodman, 1996). While the connection between specific symbolic content or elements in art expressions and emotional disorders has not been reliable, art-based assessment has demonstrated its usefulness with certain populations. The SDT has generated data indicating that it may be helpful in detecting depression (Silver, 2003). There has also been some research on the characteristics of children's human figure drawings related to emotional disorders, trauma, and abuse (Malchiodi, 1998b). Art-based assessment is employed in the field of forensics, particularly in establishing the existence of child physical and sexual abuse (Cohen-Liebman, 2002, 2003; Datillio, 2002), although verbal disclosure is still necessary to corroborate drawings as evidence.

APPROACHES TO PRACTICE

A variety of approaches to art therapy have been identified, including the psychoanalytic, object relations, cognitive-behavioral, humanistic, and developmental schools. Rubin (2001) identifies numerous approaches, and demonstrates that art therapy has been integrated with many well-known theories of psychotherapy. A recent survey conducted by the American Art Therapy Association indicates that most art therapists practice art therapy from a psychodynamic perspective, which includes psychoanalytic, object relations, and Jungian approaches (Elkins & Stovall, 2000). A high percentage of respondents indicated that they are "eclectic" in their approach, meaning that they incorporated several theoretical constructs in their work, depending on client needs and goals for treatment.

However, art therapists are not the only clinicians who use art expression in assessment and intervention. Many approaches have come from outside the field of art therapy—for example, from the fields of counseling, social work, psychology, and marriage and family therapy. Selekman (1997) uses drawing with children and families from a solution-focused approach to both verbal and experiential intervention. Freeman, Epston, and Lobovits (1997) see the value of art expression in narrative work with children, observing that children tell stories through images because verbal language is not always their preferred method of communication. Gladding (1998) has delineated the application of creative arts therapies, including art therapy, in the field of professional counseling. Finally, Riley, a marriage and family therapist and an art therapist, underscores the value of art expression in a variety of family therapy approaches including the strategic, the systemic, the narrative, and the solution-focused methods (Riley & Malchiodi, 2003; Riley, 2003).

To help the reader understand how art expression is integrated with approaches to therapy, three approaches that have dominated clinical practice of art therapy are briefly described in the following sections. For more specific information on other approaches to art therapy, see *Handbook of Art Therapy* (Malchiodi, 2003).

PSYCHOANALYTIC AND ANALYTIC APPROACHES

Psychoanalytic theory and analytic psychology have historically influenced the practice of art therapy, especially during the field's early development. Naumburg, for example, established the importance of clients' spontaneous drawings as representations and projections of their unconscious thoughts and feelings. In this sense, client-created images serve as a way to understand what is not consciously recognized through verbal associations to pictures. Edith Kramer (2001), another art therapist recognized for her contributions to the field, proposed that art expression served as a source of sublimation of aggression and other negative behaviors, thoughts, and feelings. Levick (1983) proposed that art expression is useful in identifying an individual's defense mechanisms, while Winnicott (1971) considered art a transitional object. These practitioners' observations echo psychoanalytic thinking and provide a rationale for why psychodynamic theories support art therapy.

Carl Jung's theories of archetypes and the collective unconscious also informed the analytic approach that has been popular within the field of art therapy. In using this approach, therapists emphasize the content of dreams and fantasies, helping the client to explore, amplify, and illuminate possible meanings.

While many psychoanalytic concepts have been incorporated into art therapy practice, the following have been the most influential:

- *Transference.* Simply defined, *transference* is the client's unconscious projection of feelings onto the therapist. Transference in art therapy is manifested not only through the therapist–client relationship, but also through the art expression. In other words, the art expression may also become the focus of transference and a client may react to the process of art making and to the therapist as a provider of art materials and creative activity. Finally, the content of art expression may reflect unspoken feelings about the therapist; for example, unexpressed anxiety or anger toward the therapist might surface in a drawing or painting and may become a vehicle for discussion and further intervention.
- *Spontaneous expression.* Spontaneous art expression is image making that is nondirective—that is, the person chooses what to create without direction from the therapist. Psychoanalytic and analytic approaches to art therapy are strongly connected to the idea that spontaneous art expression provides access to the unconscious in a fashion similar to that of free association. A popular technique used in art therapy is the scribble drawing, in which the individual is instructed to create a scribble and then look for images within the lines of the scribble. After images are found, the person might further articulate them with color and additional features and then make verbal associations to describe the figures or objects created. Winnicott's (1971) "squiggle game," and the "scribble technique" (Cane, 1951; Naumburg, 1966) are examples of this impromptu approach.
- *Active imagination.* Active imagination is a technique described by Jung as a way to release creativity within the individual through dreams and fantasy as the vehicles. In this process, an individual is encouraged to observe those internal images, allowing them to change and emerge while carefully attending to what is experienced. Art expression, in and of itself, is considered by some practitioners to be a form of active imagination because in art expression images arise spontaneously. Additionally, one can continue to explore an image through making additional images in response to it or using the process of active imagination to amplify it through mental imagery.

• *Transitional space and transitional objects.* Object relations theory offers two concepts that are of particular interest to art therapy: transitional space and transitional objects (Winnicott, 1953). Art making as well as play activity are considered transitional spaces because they are ways to bridge subjective and objective realities and to practice attachment and relationship. Art expression is believed to be somewhat of a "holding environment" within which object relations between therapist and client can emerge and develop. Additionally, art products can become transitional objects that may become imbued with meaning beyond what they actually are. In other words, a person may make a clay figure of a lost relative, symbolically evoking that individual and the unresolved trauma of separation and loss. Art expression may be a transitional object between therapy sessions, serving as a symbol in the absence of the therapist.

HUMANISTIC APPROACHES

Humanistic psychology, the third force in psychology, has greatly influenced the field of art therapy. Garai (2001) believes that the process of art making is an opportunity for self-actualization through self-expression and self-transcendence, underscoring the idea that creativity is part of the human proclivity to achieve wellness. Most humanistic approaches to art therapy emphasize transforming troublesome emotions, behaviors, and experiences through authentic expression as opposed to eliminating or curing them.

While there are several specific humanistic approaches to art therapy, person-centered and Gestalt approaches have been the most widely delineated. Natalie Rogers (1999), an expressive arts therapist and the daughter of Carl Rogers, has observed that active and empathetic listening underscore the person-centered approach. Additionally, because visual art or other art forms are central to the experience, the therapist has the opportunity to actively and empathetically "see" what the person is conveying. It is not the interpretation of art expression, but careful attention to what the person is communicating, that is important. Therefore, a therapist taking this approach facilitates the individual's exploration by reflecting what has been conveyed and asking for further clarification to deepen both the therapist's and the client's understanding. Art expression adds another dimension that enhances the individual's ability to communicate and serves as a nonverbal modality for understanding the person.

Gestalt therapy has also been used as a framework for humanistic art therapy. The word *Gestalt* refers to the whole form or configuration that is greater than the sum of its parts. In a Gestalt approach to art therapy, the individual, the therapist, and the art expression are part of the overall Gestalt. Because Gestalt therapy is an action-oriented approach, therapists who apply this theory believe that through sensory–motor activation, there is recognition and clarification of problems. Zinker (1977) and Rhyne (1995) have written most extensively about Gestalt art therapy. They both underscore how creative activities in therapy can be helpful in expressing personal meaning and achieving insight.

Gestalt art therapy not only incorporates art expression, but also often includes sound and music, making it similar to an integrated approach (see Chapter 9 for more information on integrated approaches). For example, a therapist taking this approach might ask a person to draw a line or shape to represent a feeling (Figure 2.1), and then ask the individual to make a sound or movement that describes the line or shape. If working with a group, the therapist may direct each of the participants to become one of the elements in a group mural or drawing and use movement or dramatic enactment to characterize his or her element. A Gestalt approach to art therapy is appropriate for people who are capable of self-direction and self-motivation because, while the therapist directs the session, it is the person who is ultimately responsible for making meaning and achieving insight.

DEVELOPMENTAL ART THERAPY

Most art therapy, especially art therapy with children, at least partly employs a developmental approach. Many therapists integrate a variety of developmental frameworks in their work, including the psychosexual (Freud, 1905/1962), the psychosocial (Erikson, 1963), and the object relations (Mahler, Pine, & Bergman, 1975) approaches. Developmental art therapy, however, is often informed by the stages of normal artistic development in children (Lowenfeld, 1957; Golumb, 1990) and their cognitive development (Piaget, 1959).

A developmental approach, along with other strategies, is commonly used with children because both the art product and the process of art making reflect aspects of human development. However, while this approach is used primarily with children, it is also valuable in therapy with adults who have experienced emotional stress or trauma. Art

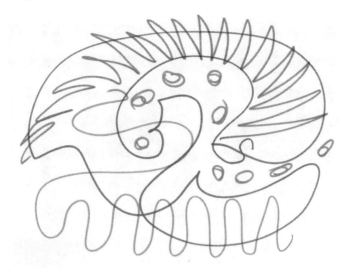

FIGURE 2.1. Drawing of lines and shapes as stimulus for movement and sound.

making in therapy with adults can evoke early sensory experiences and symbolic expression found throughout the stages of artistic development. Moreover, art expressions made by people of all ages can be considered from a developmental perspective (Malchiodi, Kim, & Choi, 2003).

In order to understand developmental art therapy, a working knowledge of the characteristics of normal artistic development is necessary. Table 2.1 provides an overview of basic characteristics for each stage and approximate age ranges. (Note: Most of the research on children's artistic development has been on how children draw; less attention has been given to other art modalities such as work with clay.) While there is individual variation, most children pass through these stages in a sequential manner and with recognizable milestones in their art expressions.

In a developmental approach, assessment ignores symbolic content to focus on a comparison of the child's artistic expression to what is normal for that age group. The therapist may also use developmental stages as a framework for evaluating motor, cognitive, or social skills. For example, the therapist might ask, Does an adolescent with moderate retardation make appropriate contact with the therapist? Does a child with autism have age-appropriate skills in using tools and materials? In a de-

TABLE 2.1. Stages of Artistic Expression

Stage I: Scribbling	18 months–3 years	During this stage the very first marks are made by a child on paper. At first there is little control of the motions that are used to make the scribble; accidental results occur and the line quality of these early drawings varies greatly.

As motor skills improve scribbles include repeated motions, making horizontal or longitudinal lines, circular shapes, and assorted dots, marks, and other forms. At this stage there is also not much conscious use of color (i.e., the color is used for enjoyment without specific intentions) and drawing is enjoyed for the kinesthetic experience it provides. Limited attention span and not much narrative about the art product. |
| 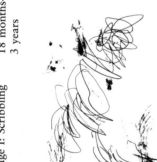 | | |
| Stage II: Basic forms | 3–4 years | Children may still make scribbles at this age, but they also become more involved in naming and inventing stories about them. The connection of one's marks on paper to the world around him or her occurs. Children want to talk about their drawings, even if they appear to adults as unidentifiable scribbles. Attention span is still limited and concentration is restricted. Meanings for images change; a child may start a scribble drawing by saying "this is my mommy," only to quickly label it as something else soon after.

Other configurations emerge at this time, including the mandala, a circular shape, design, or pattern and combinations of basic forms and shapes such as triangles, circles, crosses, squares, and rectangles. These forms are the precursors of human figures and other objects, the milestone in the next stage. |
| 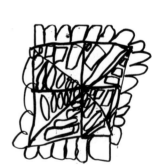 | | |

Stage III: Human forms and beginning schema   4–6 years

The major milestone of this stage is the emergence of rudimentary human figures, often called tadpoles, cephlapods, and prototypes. These human figures are often primitive and sometimes quite charming.

There is still a subjective use of color at this stage, although some children may begin to associate color in their drawings with what they perceive to be in the environment (e.g., leaves are green). Children of this age are more interested in drawing the figure or object than the color of it. Also, there is no conscious approach to composition or design, and children may place objects throughout a page without concern for a groundline or relationships to size. A figure may float freely across the page, at the top or sides, and some things may appear upside down because children are not concerned with direction or relationship of objects.

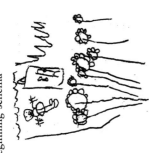

Stage IV: Development of a visual schema   6–9 years

Children rapidly progress in their artistic abilities during this stage. The first and foremost is the development of visual symbols or schema for human figures, animals, houses, trees, and other objects in the environment. Many of these symbols are fairly standard, such as a particular way to depict a head with a circle, hairstyles, arms and legs, a tree with a brown trunk and green top; a yellow sun in the upper corner of the page; and a house with a triangular, pitched roof. Color is used objectively and sometimes rigidly (e.g., all leaves must be the same color green). There is the development of a baseline (a groundline upon which objects sit) and often a skyline (a blue line across the top the drawing to indicate the sky). During these years children also draw see-through or x-ray pictures (such as cut-away images of a house, where one can see everything inside) and attempt beginning perspective by placing more distant objects higher on the drawing page.

It is normal at this age to use variations in size to emphasize importance; for example, children may depict themselves as bigger than the house or tree in the same drawing, if they wish to emphasize the figure. Or a child depicting a person throwing a ball may draw a much longer arm than usual.

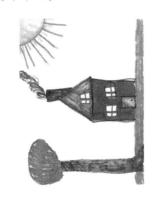

(continued)

TABLE 2.1. (*continued*)

Stage V: Realism	9–12 years	At this stage, children become interested in depicting what they perceive to be realistic elements in their drawings. This includes the first attempts at perspective; children no longer draw a simple baseline but instead draw the ground meeting the sky to create depth. There is a more accurate depiction of color in nature (e.g., leaves can be many different colors rather than just one shade of green), and the human figure is more detailed and differentiated in gender characteristics (e.g., more details in hair, clothing, and build).
		At this stage, children begin to become more conventional in their art expressions and are more literal because they want to achieve a "photographic effect" in their renditions. They may also make drawings of cartoon or comic strip characters in order to imitate an adult-like quality in their pictures. In this stage children have increasing technical abilities and enjoy exploring new materials and can work on more detailed, complicated art expressions.
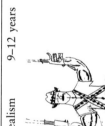		
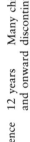		
Stage VI: Adolescence	12 years and onward	Many children (and adults) never reach this stage of artistic development because they may discontinue drawing or making art at around the age of 10 or 11 due to other interests. However, by the age of 13, children who have continued to make art or have art training will be able to use perspective more accurately and effectively in their drawings, will include greater detail in their work, will have increasing mastery of materials, will be more attentive to color and design, and will be able to create abstract images.
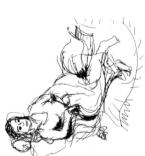		

Note. Based on the work of Lowenfeld and Brittain (1987), Gardner (1980), Kellogg (1970), and Winner (1982). Adapted from Malchiodi (1998b). Copyright 1998 by Cathy A. Malchiodi. Adapted by permission.

velopmental approach, both the art product and the process of art making are used to evaluate these and related skill areas.

In developmental art therapy, several areas in treatment planning are particularly important, including the following:

- *Sensory stimulation.* Sensory-related tasks are often part of a developmental approach. The therapist may introduce a variety of visual, motor, and interactive skills through art and play activities that involve tactile, movement, and other sensory experiences.
- *Skill acquisition.* Skill acquisition can involve learning a particular activity through sequential steps or may even include learning new behaviors and ways of interaction with the therapist and others. For example, a painting task may be introduced to help the child learn to hold a brush and eventually to dip the brush in paint; secondary goals may be to assist the child in learning how to sit at a table with other children, share materials, and interact appropriately with others.
- *Adaptation.* For some individuals, adaptation of materials and tasks is necessary. For example, an older man who has suffered a stroke may not be able to hold a pencil or a brush; the therapist may offer alternate materials or provide a way for the person to hold the drawing or painting instrument. The therapy environment may also be adapted to create consistency and eliminate disorder so that individuals can focus more easily on the activities provided.

CLINICAL APPLICATIONS WITH CHILDREN, ADULTS, GROUPS, AND FAMILIES

Art Therapy with Children

While art therapy is used with individuals of all ages, clinicians often think of its clinical application to children. In fact, most therapists who work with children use some sort of art or play because children, especially young ones, are often more comfortable expressing themselves through action rather than through words. For children who have experienced severe emotional trauma, loss, or abuse, making drawings, paintings, or other art forms is preferable to talking about that which is difficult to articulate or uncomfortable to share verbally. Art, like play and other expressive modalities, becomes a representation of the child's inner world of unspoken thoughts, feelings, and experiences.

Art therapy has been applied to a variety of child populations, including those with psychiatric, behavioral, and medical disorders (Malchiodi, 1998c). Recently, the application of art therapy with children who have posttraumatic stress disorder (PTSD), after experiencing family violence, abuse, or traumatic loss, has received attention. Drawing and other forms of creative expression have been successfully used with child survivors of adults killed in the terrorist attacks of September 11, 2001, in the United States, proving to be one of few ways to reach children's fears, anxiety, and other sequelae of these traumatic events. In these and similar cases, art therapy is particularly effective because of the sensory nature of trauma—in the case of the terrorist attacks, many children were repeatedly exposed to violent and frightening images on television (Figure 2.2). In a similar fashion, art has been used as a therapeutic intervention with children who have experienced school shootings, witnessed homicides, or experienced the death of a loved one through accidents or natural disasters (Steele, 2003). The following brief case example illustrates how art expression is used with a child who has experienced trauma.

Janie, a 6-year-old girl, was admitted along with her mother to a long-term shelter for homeless families. The apartment Janie lived in was destroyed in a fire along with all their possessions. Janie and her mother were brought to the shelter by social services because they had no relatives to go to and little or no financial resources to live on in the short term.

In the initial session, the therapist showed Janie the art and play therapy room and suggested that she might like to make something with the art supplies. The therapist introduced Janie to the materials available for her to use: felt markers and colored pencils for drawing, an easel with tempera paints for painting, and an assortment of clay for making objects. In offering Janie these three materials with which to create, the therapist hoped to evaluate the child's developmental abilities through a Kramer Evaluation (previously described in the section on art-based assessment) and to see what themes surfaced in Janie's artwork. In response, Janie chose to make a small drawing of "a little girl standing outside" (Figure 2.3). She later told the therapist that she did not want to use the paint or clay because she was afraid of "making a mess." Janie used the drawing materials in a very careful manner, obsessively covering felt markers with their caps and continually talking about her worries about spilling paint or getting clay on her clothes. In contrast to most children of her age, Janie seemed inhibited and somewhat fearful

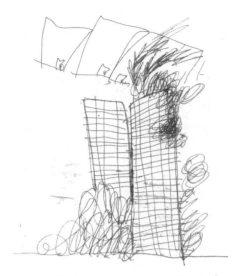

FIGURE 2.2. Drawing by child in response to terrorist attacks on Twin Towers in New York City.

about art making and seemed to lack the sense of playfulness appropriate to her stage of development. Her repetitive behaviors may also have reflected her traumatic stress: many children who experience posttraumatic stress symptoms display repetitive actions in art and play after a significant crisis or loss.

In a subsequent session and after establishing a rapport with Janie, the therapist asked her if she could draw a picture of "what happened" when the fire burnt down the apartment building. Janie quickly drew a picture of herself and her mother standing together crying in front of a mass of black lines that she identified as what was left of their "home after the fire burnt it" (Figure 2.4). As the therapist began to refer to the drawing and asked Janie to tell her more, the activity generated more verbalization about the details of Janie's experiences as well as her fears after the event. She explained to the therapist that she had lost her favorite stuffed bear and wondered out loud about a neighbor's cat that lived in the building, expressing fears that it had died in the fire. When asked if she would like to draw any other worries she had, Janie quickly drew a picture of the shelter and expressed to the therapist her anxiety that the shelter might "catch on fire if someone smoked a cigarette or didn't turn off the stove." Her drawings facilitated expression of feelings, thoughts,

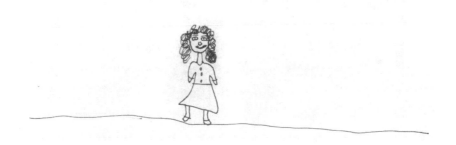

FIGURE 2.3. Janie's drawing of "a little girl standing outside."

and beliefs and provided the therapist with an understanding of Janie's feelings of fright and lack of control.

In other sessions the therapist encouraged Janie to use art and play materials to express more about the fire and any other feelings she had about what happened. As Janie felt more comfortable and less preoccupied with worries, the therapist was able to introduce her to work in clay and paint and helped Janie to engage in playful experiences with these materials. Janie began to feel more confident and in control in contrast to her initial inability to work with clay or paint, materials that are not easily controlled.

For Janie, art expression was an effective way to help her convey her feelings, particularly worry and fear, to the therapist, as well as to communicate aspects of the trauma that she may not have spontaneously verbalized. While art therapy has been successfully used in the treatment of trauma in children, it is useful with many disorders of children as well as adolescents. ADHD (Safran, 2002) and autism (Gabriels, 2003) are two disorders that are particularly suited to art therapy because developmental, behavioral, and emotional issues can be addressed through creative activity. Adolescents are also particularly good candidates for art therapy because artistic expression is often a way to reach both those individuals who are withdrawn and those who are resistant to verbal therapy. It provides a creative way to communicate without words that teenagers may find preferable. Additionally, family art therapy (see below for more information) often becomes part of the treatment because working with parents and siblings may be important to successful intervention.

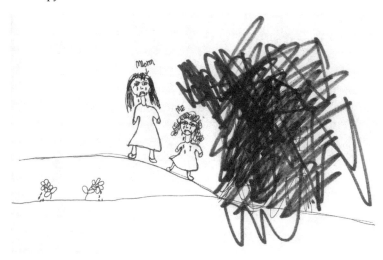

FIGURE 2.4. Janie's drawing of her mother and herself crying in front of their home (mass of black lines).

Art Therapy with Adults

In therapy with adults, art expression serves as a form of nonverbal communication of feelings, thoughts, and worldviews and provides an opportunity to explore problems, strengths, and possibilities for change. The creative process of art making can be applied to work with adults throughout the lifespan, from young adulthood to well into old age. The major portion of art therapy's foundations as a field derives from early work with adults hospitalized for psychiatric disorders. Naumburg's ideas about spontaneous drawings and approaches to treatment were formulated from her work with adult patients.

Art therapy is particularly useful with adult clients who may be resistant to verbal therapy or who may, for personal or cultural reasons, find it difficult to talk about themselves or problems. An art expression, whether a simple stick figure, a photocollage, or a more elaborate painting, is something that both the client and the therapist can view and discuss, taking the attention off the client for the moment. In contrast to work with children, when working with adults a therapist can capitalize on art expressions as a way to help the client clarify experiences, reframe problems, and experiment with possible solutions through drawing or other creative activities.

Art therapy with adults has often taken a psychoanalytic approach, but also has been integrated with more contemporary theories of intervention. For example, cognitive-behavioral approaches to art therapy are currently popular because art expression can easily be applied within these constructs. In work with adult clients, Rozum and Malchiodi (2003, p. 76) suggest the following interventions that blend art tasks with cognitive-behavioral therapy:

• *Make an image of a "stressor."* Identifying stressors that trigger negative feelings is basic to a cognitive-behavioral approach. The client may be encouraged to make an image of the stressful event that contributes to negative self-talk or to keep a visual journal of situations that initiate negative behaviors.

• *Make an image of "how I can prepare for a stressor."* The client may be asked to create an image of "what I do to meet a challenging situation." For example, if public speaking is a trigger for anxious feelings, the therapist may encourage the individual to make a picture with images that illustrate positive ways to address the situation.

• *Make an image of "step-by-step management" of a problem.* Therapists who work from a cognitive-behavioral approach often help individuals to break down a problem into components or steps to a solution. Making a picture or series of pictures to illustrate how a problem can be addressed through more manageable parts may be helpful for some clients.

• *Create imagery for stress reduction.* The act of creating images can serve as a "time-out" from negative thinking or behaviors and may be useful in inducing the relaxation response. Therapists may also suggest to clients that they collect images of soothing pictures from magazines or other sources and make a collage or visual journal to induce positive thoughts when needed.

Therapists who use cognitive-behavioral approaches often prescribe homework; in the case of art therapy, drawing or other art activities may be suggested between sessions. The following brief case example illustrates some of the principles of a cognitive-behavioral approach to art therapy with an adult.

Marsha, a 29-year-old graduate student, was having difficulties with her studies because of stress. Occasionally, she had panic attacks, particularly when she became overwhelmed with completing course assignments or preparing for an exam. Marsha sought the help of a therapist when she had a particularly bad panic attack during a midterm exam and a friend had to take her to the hospital because Marsha felt short of breath and reported heart palpitations. On a subsequent examination, her physician found nothing physically wrong with Marsha and suggested that she take an antidepressant that was helpful for the panic disorder and another medication as needed for anxiety. He also recommended that some counseling sessions might increase the effectiveness of medication and that cognitive-behavioral therapy was one approach shown to be effective with the type of anxiety she was experiencing.

During their initial meeting, after obtaining a patient history, the therapist asked Marsha to draw on a simple body outline what it was like to have a panic attack and what it would be like to be "panic-free" (Figures 2.5 and 2.6). While Marsha was drawing these images the therapist asked her to describe any specific feelings or sensations in her body that she had during an episode of anxiety. The therapist also asked Marsha if there were any particular thoughts she had during an attack. Marsha reported that she often told herself that she must be "crazy," followed by "I feel like I am going to faint or die."

The goal in this approach is to help the individual learn self-care and preventative measures and to provide the person with the education and skills necessary to recognize and overcome anxiety. In helping Marsha to understand what her panic felt like in her body through drawing and any automatic thoughts she had during an attack, the therapist began to help her understand how her perceptions of body sensations and negative self-talk could escalate her panic. In addition, the therapist prescribed "homework" in the form of a drawing journal in which Marsha was asked to draw images of her feelings between sessions and keep a record of how she responded to cognitive-behavioral exercises she practiced between sessions and psychopharmacological intervention. The therapist also suggested some breathing exercises and drawing activities to help Marsha reduce stress when she felt herself becoming panicked or having negative thoughts that could lead to anxiety or discomfort.

In brief, a cognitive-behavioral approach to art therapy may use art tasks for a variety of reasons: to help identify the client's reasons for coming to therapy, to understand how the client perceives art therapy as a form of treatment, and to encourage the client to become an active participant in therapy. Art expression is also used to help the individual "literally" reframe troublesome emotions or experiences as well as to create new solutions with the help of the therapist.

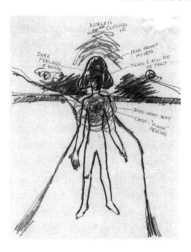

FIGURE 2.5. Marsha's body outline showing "what a panic attack feels like."

Art Therapy with Groups

Art therapy, like other forms of treatment, often occurs in hospitals, outpatient clinics, shelters, community agencies, and other settings where therapy or counseling takes place in groups. Group art therapy, like any group therapy, creates the opportunity for communication and interac-

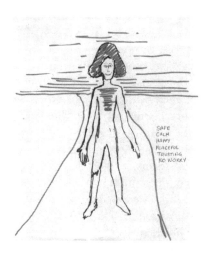

FIGURE 2.6. Marsha's body outline showing herself as "panic-free."

tions with others. This communication and interaction may be directed toward a specific theme, such as substance abuse or bereavement, or it may be less formal, such as in a therapist-facilitated studio where people come to make art and share their experiences with others in a supportive environment.

Group art therapy offers some special qualities that have "curative potential" for its participants. Yalom, a psychiatrist known for his work with groups, believes there are "curative factors" found in groups; many of these are present within group art therapy (Yalom, 1995). These include *instilling hope* through group support and mutual sharing of problem solving and recovery; *interaction* through conjoint work on group art activities or through sharing one's art expressions with others during a session; *universality* through learning that one's problems are similar and through seeing that others express similar universal meanings; and *altruism* through reinforcing positive support and exchange through creative activities (Malchiodi, 1998a). These curative characteristics apply to most group art therapy. A therapist may capitalize on one or more of them through experiential work.

In many art therapy groups, the therapist takes on an active leadership role, determining themes and directives for the group. The therapist may design group art activities with particular goals in mind or as the group progresses or presents new problems or themes. For example, in working with a group of breast cancer survivors in initial sessions, a therapist may explore ideas and issues with participants in order to develop goals and specific activities addressing medical treatment, issues of loss and grief, and social support. Group art therapy might begin with an opening discussion or warm-up activity, followed by a directive for individual or conjoint art making, and ending with a postexperiential discussion. As the group progress, the therapist and participants may make adjustments to the group art activities as issues emerge or interests change. In contrast, some group art therapy is nondirective and participants make art of their own choosing. Goals may focus on creating an atmosphere for interaction, creative expression, and art making as a form of therapy in and of itself.

The most important advantage of using art expression within a framework of group therapy may be its ability to make the group process visible. Riley (2001) notes that "when creative thoughts and opportunities emerge in the group process, it is essential to anchor them in an observable expression" (p. 4). Art expression is a way to make interpersonal processes tangible and can visually record a moment in time or a pattern of interaction.

Art Therapy with Families

Family art therapy is based on one or more of the many theoretical principles commonly used in the field of marriage and family therapy. There are a variety of art therapy approaches to work with families, including strategic, systemic, structural, solution-focused, narrative, and others (Riley & Malchiodi, 2003). Art expression is particularly useful with families because it offers family members a way to visually portray their feelings, perspectives, and worldviews. It also allows every generation to have an equal voice through images—even the youngest child can participate actively in treatment. Family art therapy can enhance communication among family members and may help them to convey, both through the process and the content of art making, family patterns of interaction and behavior (Riley & Malchiodi, 2003).

A family art therapy approach can also be employed with individual clients, just as marriage and family therapy is often used with a single client seen outside a family or couple. For example, creating a drawing or collage about one's family allows an individual to illustrate family roles, issues, and problems in one's family of origin. Additionally, a creative genogram, using color and symbols to represent one's family members, can help both therapist and client to identify patterns of behavior, commonly held beliefs, and family stories passed from one generation to the next. The following case example illustrates family art therapy from a solution-focused, strategic approach.

The Jimenez family had been to several therapists over the last year and felt discouraged that "no one was able to help them with their problem." Maria, 28 years old, initially sought therapy at a local agency for her son, Jose, 9 years old, because he "does not follow her rules, had tantrums, and does not get along with Chia" (his younger sister, 6 years old). Jose's school counselor recommended the initial course of therapy because he was having behavioral problems at school and was thought to have ADHD. A therapist at the agency referred the case to my practice so that Jose would have both individual and family art and play therapy.

Ten days after an initial session to establish goals and objectives, I met with the Jimenez family (Maria; Juan, her husband; and Jose; Chia did not attend because of illness) for their second family therapy session. In order to obtain additional information on the family and their families of origin, this session was devoted to doing "creative genograms"— each family member created a quick drawing using colors, shapes, and/ or images (such as stick figures or doodles) to depict individuals in the family. For example, a blue circle might be used to represent someone, a yellow squiggle to represent someone else, and so forth (see Figure 2.7).

From listening and responding to these art expressions, I co-constructed a traditional genogram (in pencil) with the family that helped me to more clearly understand their family of origin as well as current relationships between family members and families of origin. The Jimenez family responded positively to this activity and enjoyed telling more about their family's story, including their move to the United States, memories of Mexico, Maria's and Juan's meeting in high school, their eventual marriage, and the births of Jose and Chia. I learned several facts that were previously not disclosed. First, Jose's birth had been a difficult one and Maria worried that her difficult pregnancy and labor "caused Jose's ADHD." Juan and Maria also reported that Maria's conflict with her sister was a significant source of stress to them and Maria's mother; Maria, Juan, and Maria's mother had not spoken to her sister for 6 months and before that communication had been strained and conflict-ridden. Maria also confided that her father's accidental death might have been caused by his addiction to alcohol; he had been drinking on the evening of the accident and drove his car into a ravine. She volunteered that her sister's drug addiction was similar to their father's

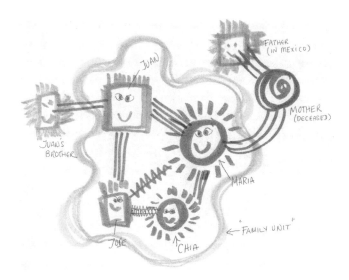

FIGURE 2.7. Maria's creative genogram.

alcohol addiction and that she was both sad and angry that her sister might die from her addiction "in a foolish way, such as an accident."

The next session focused on helping the family investigate and define how Jose's ADHD was influencing the Jimenez family. In this session, I took a narrative approach (White & Epston, 1990) and helped the family "externalize" Jose's problem as something that "was pushing this family around." I explained that while Jose may be the one with ADHD, ADHD affected everyone in the family, not just Jose. I wondered out loud about how we could "maybe stop ADHD from pushing Jose, Maria, Juan, and Chia around all the time" because ADHD "was giving Jose and his family a really hard time." I asked each person to try to draw a self-image of what "ADHD looked like when it was pushing you around." In brief, these quick images generated a discussion about how Jose felt when he had un-controllable outbursts, was aggressive, or was destructive. Maria and Juan were able to more clearly describe how they felt when Jose's ADHD trig-gered emotional outbursts within the family and what specific aspects of ADHD escalated into arguments, yelling, and power struggles. From externalizing ADHD in this manner, we were able to come up with some specific behavioral goals for Jose and ways for the family to "respond to ADHD" in a more effective manner.

While additional sessions and interventions involved assisting this family in resolving their problems and achieving their goals, the intro-duction of creative expression helped this family to communicate issues and feelings to each other. For Jose and Chia, hands-on activities al-lowed them to feel like active participants in treatment in contrast to the verbally oriented family therapy they had experienced in the past. Juan commented that "this kind of therapy is actually fun and it is has been a long time since we were all able to laugh and play together." Maria was surprised that "using pictures and drawings helped her to remember things about her family" that she had forgotten and used some of the ac-tivities with Jose and Chia at home between sessions. In summary, the introduction of art activities helped this family to express their feelings and offered them a modality through which they could confront and re-solve their problems in new and creative ways.

CONCLUSION

Art therapy is an action-oriented modality offering individuals of all ages possibilities for communication, enhancing verbal exchange, and literally letting the therapist and client "see" things from a different perspective. Like other expressive therapies, it also provides a process that engages the senses and complements traditional "talk" methods. Images can convey the thoughts, feelings, and experiences of the people who create them, but the most important aspect of art therapy is the facilitation of individuals' discovery of personal meaning for their art expressions. Whether used as a primary therapy or as an adjunct to verbal approaches, art therapy offers a variety of avenues for children, adults, families, and groups to overcome emotional distress, reframe problems, resolve conflicts, achieve insights, change behaviors, and increase an overall sense of well-being.

REFERENCES

American Art Therapy Association. (1996). *Mission statement.* Mundelein, IL: Author.

Buck, J. (1986). *House–Tree–Person technique: Revised manual.* Beverly Hills, CA: Western Psychological Services.

Burns, R., & Kaufman, S. (1972). *Actions, styles, and symbols in Kinetic Family Drawings (KFD): An interpretative manual.* New York: Brunner/Mazel.

Cane, F. (1951). *The artist in each of us.* Craftsbury Common, VT: Art Therapy.

Cohen-Liebman, M. (2002). Art therapy. In A. Giardino & E. Giardino (Eds.), *Recognition of child abuse for the mandated reporter* (pp. 227–258). St. Louis, MO: G. W. Medical.

Cohen-Liebman, M. S. (2003). Drawings in forensic investigations of child sexual abuse. In C. A. Malchiodi (Ed.), *Handbook of art therapy* (pp. 167–180). New York: Guilford Press.

Councill, T. (2003). Medical art therapy with children. In C. A. Malchiodi (Ed.), *Handbook of art therapy* (pp. 207–219). New York: Guilford Press.

Dattilio, F. (2002). *Mental health experts: Roles and qualifications for court.* Mechanicsburg: Pennsylvania Bar Institute.

Elkins, D., & Stovall, K. (2000). American Art Therapy Association, Inc.: 1998–1999 Membership Survey Report. *Art Therapy: Journal of the American Art Therapy Association, 17,* 41–46.

Erikson, E. (1963). *Childhood and society.* New York: Norton.

Freeman, J., Epston, D., & Lobovits, D. (1997). *Playful approaches to serious problems: Narrative therapy with children and their families.* New York: Norton.

Freud, S. (1953). Three essays on the theory of sexuality. In J. Strachey (Ed. and Trans.), *The standard edition of the complete psychological works of Sigmund Freud* (Vol. 7, pp. 123–245). London: Hogarth Press. (Original work published 1905)

Gabriels, R. L. (2003). Art therapy with children who have autism and their families. In C. A. Malchiodi (Ed.), Handbook of art therapy (pp. 193–206). New York: Guilford Press.

Gantt, L., & Tabone, C. (2003). The Formal Elements Arts Therapy Scale and "Draw a Person Picking an Apple from a Tree." In C. A. Malchiodi (Ed.), Handbook of art therapy (pp. 420–427). New York: Guilford Press.

Garai, J. (2001). A humanistic approach to art therapy. In J. Rubin (Ed.), Approaches to art therapy (pp. 188–207). New York: Brunner-Routledge.

Gardner, H. (1980). Artful scribbles. New York: Basic Books.

Gladding, S. (1998). Counseling as an art. Alexandria, VA: American Counseling Association.

Gladding, S., & Newsome, D. (2003). Art in counseling. In C. A. Malchiodi (Ed.), Handbook of art therapy (pp. 243–253). New York: Guilford Press.

Golumb, G. (1990). The child's creation of the pictorial world. Berkeley and Los Angeles: University of California Press.

Gross, J., & Haynes, H. (1998). Drawing facilitates children's verbal reports of emotionally laden events. Journal of Experimental Psychology, 4, 163–179.

Kellogg, R. (1970). Analyzing children's art. Palo Alto, CA: Mayfield.

Koppitz, E. (1968). Psychological evaluation of human figure drawings by middle school pupils. Orlando, FL: Grune & Stratton.

Kramer, E. (2001). Art as therapy: Collected papers. London: Kingsley.

Kramer, E., & Schehr, J. (1983). An art therapy evaluation session for children. American Journal of Art Therapy, 23(1), 3–12.

Levick, M. (1983). They could not talk and so they drew: Children's styles of coping and thinking. Springfield, IL: Thomas.

Lillienfeld, S., Wood, J., & Grab, H. (2000). The scientific status of projective techniques. Psychological Science in the Public Interest, 1(2), 27–66.

Lowenfeld, V. (1957). Creative and mental growth (3rd ed.). New York: Macmillan.

Lowenfeld, V., & Brittain, W. (1987). Creative and mental growth (7th ed.). New York: Macmillan.

Mahler, M., Pine, F., & Bergman, A. (1975). The psychological birth of the human infant: Symbiosis and individuation. New York: Basic Books.

Malchiodi, C. A. (1998a). The art therapy sourcebook. New York: McGraw-Hill.

Malchiodi, C. A. (1998b). Understanding children's drawings. New York: Guilford Press.

Malchiodi, C. A. (1998c). Medical art therapy with children. London: Kingsley.

Malchiodi, C. A. (1999). Medical art therapy with adults. London: Kingsley.

Malchiodi, C. A. (2000). Art therapy and computer technology. London: Kingsley.

Malchiodi, C. A. (2002). The soul's palette. Boston: Shambhala.

Malchiodi, C. A. (Ed.). (2003). Handbook of art therapy. New York: Guilford Press.

Malchiodi, C. A., Kim, D.-Y., & Choi, W. S. (2003). Developmental art therapy. In C. A. Malchiodi (Ed.), Handbook of art therapy (pp. 93–105). New York: Guilford Press.

Mills, A. (2003). The Diagnostic Drawing Series. In C. A. Malchiodi (Ed.), Handbook of art therapy (pp. 401–409). New York: Guilford Press.

Naumburg, M. (1966). *Dynamically-oriented art therapy: Its principles and practice.* New York: Grune & Stratton.

Piaget, J. (1959). *Judgment and reasoning in the child.* Patterson, NJ: Littlefield Adams.

Rhyne, J. (1995). *The Gestalt art experience.* Chicago: Magnolia Street.

Riley, S. (2001). *Group process made visible.* New York: Brunner-Routledge.

Riley, S. (2003). Art therapy with couples. In C. A. Malchiodi (Ed.), *Handbook of art therapy* (pp. 387–398). New York: Guilford Press.

Riley, S., & Malchiodi, C. A. (2003). *Family art therapy.* In C. A. Malchiodi (Ed.), *Handbook of art therapy* (pp. 362–374). New York: Guilford Press.

Rogers, N. (1999). *The creative connection: Expressive arts as healing.* Palo Alto, CA: Science and Behavior Books.

Rozum, A. L., & Malchiodi, C. A. (2003). Cognitive-behavioral approaches. In C. A. Malchiodi (Ed.), *Handbook of art therapy* (pp. 72–81). New York: Guilford Press.

Rubin, J. (2001). *Approaches to art therapy: Theory and techniques* (2nd ed.). New York: Brunner-Routledge.

Safran, D. (2002). *Art therapy and ADHD.* London: Kingsley.

Selekman, M. D. (1997). *Solution-focused therapy with children.* New York: Guilford Press.

Silver, R. (2002). *Three art assessments.* New York: Brunner-Routledge.

Silver, R. A. (2003). The Silver Drawing Test of Cognition and Emotion. In C. A. Malchiodi (Ed.), *Handbook of art therapy* (pp. 410–419). New York: Guilford Press.

Steele, W. (2003). Using drawings in short-term trauma resolution. In C. A. Malchiodi (Ed.), *Handbook of art therapy* (pp. 139–151). New York: Guilford Press.

Vick, R. M. (2003). A brief history of art therapy. In C. A. Malchiodi (Ed.), *Handbook of art therapy* (pp. 5–15). New York: Guilford Press.

Wadeson, H. (2002). The anti-assessment devil's advocate. *Art Therapy: Journal of the American Art Therapy Association, 19*(4), 168–170.

White, M., & Epston, D. (1990). *Narrative means to therapeutic ends.* New York: Norton.

Wieser, J. (1993). *Phototherapy techniques.* San Francisco: Jossey-Bass.

Williams, K., Agell, G., Gantt, L., & Goodman, R. (1996). Art-based diagnosis: Fact or fantasy? *American Journal of Art Therapy, 35*(1), 9–31.

Winner, E. (1982). *Invented worlds: The psychology of the arts.* Cambridge, MA: Harvard University.

Winnicott, D. (1953). Transitional objects and transitional phenomena. *International Journal of Psychiatry, 34,* 89–97.

Winnicott, D. (1971). *Therapeutic consultation on child psychiatry.* New York: Basic Books.

Yalom, I. (1995). *The theory and practice of group psychotherapy* (4th ed.). New York: Basic Books.

Zinker, J. (1978). *Creative process in Gestalt therapy.* New York: Brunner/Mazel.

3

Music Therapy

MICHELE FORINASH

Music therapy can trace its origins to the shamans of historic times who harnessed the curative power of music to aid those suffering from a variety of maladies. Today music therapy is an internationally recognized and practiced discipline. The current definition of music therapy in the United States is "the prescribed use of music by a qualified person to effect positive change in psychological, physical, cognitive, or social functioning of individuals with health or educational problems" (available from *www.musictherapy.org*)

In the United States the origins of music therapy can be traced to post-World War II veterans hospitals. Musicians, who had long been performing in these hospitals, found that patients suffering both physically and emotionally were often responsive to music while unresponsive to other forms of engagement. The first training program began in the United States in 1944. In 1950 what is now called the American Music Therapy Association (AMTA) was founded. As of 2004 there are approximately 4,000 music therapists in the United States.

In addition to a solid national presence, music therapy has a rich international heritage. Music therapy is taught and practiced around the world, including Europe, Asia, South America, Australia, and Russia (see *www.voices.no*). There are an estimated 15,000 music therapists worldwide (Grocke, 2002).

OVERVIEW OF MUSIC THERAPY

Classification

One can find music therapists in a wide variety of settings, doing quite different types of music therapy, and practicing from diverse theoretical perspectives. Providing a classification of the major approaches is not a simple task. Bruscia (1998) defined six general areas in which music therapists practice: (1) *didactic*, primarily educational in nature, which emphasizes obtaining skills necessary for functional independent living; (2) *medical*, which focuses on restoration or maintenance of health; (3) *healing*, which is the use of the universal energy forms inherent in music for change; (4) *psychotherapeutic*, which provides clients with experiences leading to meaning and fulfillment; (5) *recreational*, which uses music for personal enjoyment; and (6) *ecological*, which focuses on promoting health in the community, family, and workplace.

Approaching classification from a different angle, Ruud (1980) categorizes music therapy practice in relation to four theories of psychology: (1) *psychodynamic*, focusing on unconscious motivations and drives; (2) *behavioral*, focusing on overt, observable behaviors; (3) *humanistic*, focusing on self-actualization and personal meaning; and (4) *transpersonal*, focusing on transcendent experiences and unity consciousness.

There are also five current international models of music therapy that represent a variety of clinical approaches. A model of music therapy is one that has a specific orientation in a theory of psychology (i.e., psychodynamic, behavioral, biomedical, humanistic, or transpersonal), has defined assessment protocols (which can be musically based), has treatment planning (with specific techniques such as improvisation), and includes evaluation. A model would therefore include "theoretical principles, clinical indications and contraindications, goals, methodological guidelines and specifications, and the characteristic use of certain procedural sequences and techniques" (Bruscia, 1998, p. 115). The five internationally recognized models are (1) *behavioral music therapy* (behavioral), (2) *Benenzon music therapy* (psychodynamic), (3) *Nordoff–Robbins music therapy* (humanistic and transpersonal), (4) *analytical music therapy* (psychodynamic), and (5) *the Bonny method of guided imagery and music* (humanistic and transpersonal).

Fundamental Philosophical Issues

Music therapy can be applied in a variety of ways. Bruscia (1998, p. 113) uses the word *method* to refer to the type of music experience the therapist provides for the client. Therapists use the following methods for purposes of assessment, treatment, and evaluation:

- *Improvisation* includes making up or improvising music, either alone or with others. Typical goals of improvisation experiences include providing nonverbal communication; promoting self-expression; exploring relationships; enhancing intimacy; acquiring group skills; encouraging creativity, spontaneity, and playfulness; stimulating the senses; and developing cognitive skills (p. 115).
- *Recreative experiences* are those in which the client and the therapist use precomposed music in treatment. They can include reproducing, performing, or interpreting musical selections. Typical goals include developing sensorimotor skills, developing time-ordered behavior, improving attention span, developing memory skills, learning specific role behaviors, and improving interactional skills (p. 116).
- *Composition experiences* focus on the creation of specific musical product. Such experiences can take the form of writing songs, lyrics, or instrumental pieces or creating audio or video projects. Typical goals include developing planning and organizing abilities, enhancing skills in problem solving, encouraging self-responsibility, and developing the ability to create an organized integrated product (p. 119).
- *Receptive experiences* are those in which the client listens to live or prerecorded music and responds either verbally or by using another art form such as drawing. Typical goals are promoting receptivity, stimulating physical responses, stimulating or relaxing the client, evoking affective states and imagery, and stimulating peak experiences (p. 121).

Another important issue in the practice of music therapy is the *role of music and words in the therapeutic process*. In some approaches the music-making process is at the forefront and is considered the agent of change; in other words, it is the experience of music that creates change in the client. For a music therapy experience to be successful or meaningful it does not have to move into a verbal discussion. This is described as *music as therapy*. In other approaches, it is the verbal processing of the music experience that leads to insight and therefore change—the experience of music becomes the stepping-stone to verbal discussion and insight. This is referred to as *music in therapy*. This discussion of music *as* therapy versus music *in* therapy in the field is ongoing. Some music therapy clinicians see their work as falling purely into one of the categories, while others use both perspectives depending on the presenting needs of the client.

Additionally, another consideration in music therapy practice is the *level of practice*. Wheeler (1983), basing her work on Wolberg (1977), has written about three levels of music therapy practice: supportive, reeducative, and reconstructive. *Supportive music therapy* is focused on restoring "individuals to an emotional equilibrium so that they can function as closely as possible to their normal levels" (1983, p. 9). *Reeducative music therapy* helps individuals to achieve awareness of their issues and helps them obtain "sufficient command of their difficulties to enable them to keep acting out impulses in check" (p. 9). *Reconstructive music therapy* focuses on changing the basic structure of the personality. This is used with individuals "whose egos are strong enough to change and who are interested enough and who are able to devote extensive time to the process" (p. 9).

Bruscia (1998) describes four levels of practice: (1) *auxiliary*, the use of music for nonmusical purposes and without a focus on the therapeutic process that leads to change; (2) *augmentative*, which augments "the education, development, healing, or therapy" (p. 168) of clients; (3) *intensive*, which focuses on the music therapist working as an equal partner with other treatment modalities; and (4) *primary*, when music therapy takes "an indispensable or singular role in meeting the main therapeutic needs of the client" (p. 170) and results in pervasive change in the client.

The process of music therapy, regardless of the therapist's philosophical orientation or the population being treated, begins with a referral from teachers, therapists, doctors, individuals (family members or friends), or clients themselves. An assessment or intake follows referral. In the assessment the therapist, either alone (if functioning as a primary therapist) or with others (if the therapist is part of a team) assesses the client and determines goals, objectives, and a specific orientation to treatment. As treatment progresses, either ongoing or periodic evaluation occurs in which the therapist evaluates the client's progress and determines the efficacy of treatment and refines treatment goals. The final step in the process is termination when the client ends music therapy treatment.

MAJOR APPROACHES TO MUSIC THERAPY

This section provides a brief discussion of several of the major approaches of music therapy.

Behavioral Music Therapy

Behavioral music therapy is the use of music to manage behavior. "The therapist uses music to increase or modify adaptive (or appropriate) behaviors and to extinguish maladaptive (or inappropriate) behaviors" (Bruscia, 1998, p. 184). According to Davis, Gfeller,and Thaut (1999), behavioral music therapy employs many of the traditional behavior modification techniques. *Positive reinforcement* is simply rewarding appropriate behavior. In a music therapy session the therapist can provide the client with a musical reward such as music lessons or listening to preferred music when the client has demonstrated an appropriate response. The response that the therapist is seeking is usually a nonmusical goal such as attending to a task for a specified period of time or other desired behavioral change.

Differential reinforcement is also used in a behavioral music therapy approach. This involves positive reinforcement for appropriate behaviors while ignoring maladaptive behaviors, thereby extinguishing the undesirable behaviors. In music therapy, this includes providing a musical reward for appropriate behaviors while disregarding inappropriate behaviors such as tantrums or acting-out.

When music is used as a reward and therefore creates a situation that is normally reinforcing for the client, the technique of "time-out" can be used. In a session where a client is engaged in an enjoyable musical activity and then shows maladaptive behaviors, the therapist can remove the client for a brief period of time. Over time this strategy is designed to decrease the maladaptive behavior. The creation of a token economy is also a useful technique in behavioral music therapy. The client can either earn, through appropriate behavior, the opportunity to engage in musical activity or can lose the privilege of engaging in music by demonstrating undesirable behavior.

This model of music therapy focuses on overt behaviors and not the actual musical activities or processes. It can be successfully applied to a variety of clinical populations. Typical goals of behavioral music therapy are to improve social skills, to improve academic skills, and to improve adaptive behaviors.

While there are no formal assessment and evaluation procedures that apply across all populations, assessment usually revolves around the following steps. The first step is to "pinpoint the behavior that is to be eliminated or established" (Madsen, 1981, p. 5), thereby setting the direction for the therapy. Next, the therapist records the client's specific behaviors. The behaviors must be measurable so that the therapist can determine when change has occurred. The subsequent step is to "consequate," which means to create contingencies or consequences for the targeted behaviors. Reinforcements used in this step can be musical, such as listening to music, playing in a group, or having a music lesson. The final step is to evaluate the outcome of the treatment (pp. 5–6).

Developmental Music Therapy

Developmental music therapy, another popular approach, is the use of music to achieve developmental goals that have been either delayed or blocked during the client's psychosocial growth. This approach is used with clients of all ages "who are encountering obstacles to developmental growth in any area (e.g., sensorimotor, cognitive, affective, interpersonal)" (Bruscia, 1998, p. 189). Edith Boxill (1985) has used developmental music therapy with individuals with developmental disabilities. Working primarily with clients who have severe delays due to disorders occurring at birth, she uses active music making with the clients as a nonverbal way of making contact. Her approach is humanistically based and focuses on affecting and enhancing "all domains of functioning—motoric, communicative, cognitive, affective, and social—always with a view to nurturing the human being as an entity, as a whole that is greater than its parts" (1985, p. 15).

Boxill considers this to be a primary treatment modality for people with developmental delays as it addresses the full scope of disabilities and delays presented by the clients. She explains that the experience of music is essentially pleasurable and therefore generates feelings of success, which then create the motivation for learning and development.

Boxill has created an in-depth assessment for work with the developmentally disabled. It includes general characteristic such as observable behaviors, physical handicaps, eye contact, and attention span; motor functioning including fine and gross motor skills, psychomotor skills, and perceptual-motor functions; communication including speech and vocal characteristics; cognitive functioning including comprehension and body awareness; affective functioning including facial expressions and range of affect; social functioning including awareness of self, others, and the environment, interaction, and participation; and specific musical behaviors such as singing on pitch and singing phrases (pp. 50–57).

Boxill uses the phrase "continuum of awareness" to describe her approach. She uses music as a way to create and enhance contact with clients to "awaken, heighten, and expand awareness of self, others, and the environment" (1985, p. 71). Music making is a vibrant and interactive process as she moves through the continuum. She usually begins treatment by mirroring or matching the client in both musical and nonmusical forms. A musical and a nonmusical here and now representation of the client–therapist interaction then follows. Finally, she creates what she terms a "contact song" (p. 75) that is either composed or improvised and serves as both a affirmation of the relationship and as a form for reciprocal communication.

Music Psychotherapy

Music psychotherapy focuses on "helping a person make those psychological changes deemed necessary or desirable to achieve well being" (Bruscia, 1998, p. 1). Bruscia lists typical goals of music psychotherapy as follows:

> greater self awareness, resolution of inner conflicts, emotional release, self-expression, changes in emotions and attitudes, improved interpersonal skills, resolution of interpersonal problems, development of healthy relationships, healing of emotional trauma, deeper insight, reality orientation, cognitive restructuring, behavior change, greater meaning and fulfillment in life, or spiritual development. (1998, p. 2)

There are a variety of ways with which music therapists approach music psychotherapy. Scheiby (1999) distinguishes between them. A Freudian-oriented music therapist would not actively play with the client, but would reflect and interpret the client's music. This type of therapist would also have responsibilities for "identifying the issue, suggesting the appropriate action method, and leading the verbal process and integration after the improvisation" (p. 264).

The Jungian music therapist would have permission to take part in the improvisation, depending on the intent. This therapist would "focus more on musical gestalts and ways of expression that can be related to as musical archetypes, such as projections of the animus/anima or identification of the musical shadow or persona, while at the same time focusing on facilitating a musical individuation process" (p. 265).

The therapist working from an object relations approach would participate in the improvisations and focus on the "client's developmental stage through the qualities of the client's music that reflect problems of symbiosis, separation and rapprochement" (p. 265). In this approach music is often used as a transitional object, echoing the ideas of Winnicott (1971).

The Gestalt-oriented therapist usually actively participates in the client's improvisation. The focus here would be on "intrapersonal and interpersonal contact with the here and now, awareness, and energy during the improvisation" (p. 265).

Analytical music therapy (AMT) as developed by Mary Priestly in the 1970s is a music-based psychotherapy approach. Clearly inspired by psychodynamic traditions, Priestly's AMT focuses on "the client's verbal processing of musical improvisation to better integrate emotions, bodily awareness, and cognitive insights" (p. 266).

Medical Music Therapy

Medical music therapy is defined as that which takes place in medical facilities. It focuses on helping clients to improve, restore, or maintain physical well-being and on the emotional issues that accompany medical treatment.

Dileo (1999) distinguishes two uses of music in medical settings: music medicine and music therapy. *Music medicine* is the use of receptive music techniques such as music listening to aid in various treatments or medical situations. Medical personnel rather than music therapists usually instigate music medicine. According to Dileo, "It often represents an attempt to provide a nonpharmacological intervention for stress, anxiety, and/or pain for the medical patient. Examples of music medicine interventions include background music in waiting rooms or other areas of the hospital/treatment environment, music programs available to the patient prior to surgery or other procedures, and vibroacoustic treatment" (1999, p. 4).

In contrast, *medical music therapy* uses a wide variety of music therapy methods such as improvising, re-creating, or composing, and is focused on the therapeutic process and the relationship between patient and therapist. Medical music therapy addresses the whole client and not just the presenting medical condition (Dileo, 1999). Within medical music therapy one can find practitioners from the variety of theoretical approaches discussed earlier (behavioral, psychodynamic, humanistic, etc.), as well as some from emerging perspectives such as a model focused on wellness.

Music therapy in the treatment of neurological disorders is a specialization within medical music therapy. *Neurological disorders* include all disorders related to injury of the brain or the nervous system including stroke, traumatic brain injury, multiple sclerosis, Alzheimer's disease, and Parkinson's disease (Tomaino, 1999, p. 115). Tomaino, working from a humanistic approach, discusses the power of music as a therapeutic tool for the neurologically impaired:

> People's experience with music throughout their lives can influence how they will respond to rhythm and sounds presented during therapy sessions. Research in neuroscience indicates there is a strong connection between the auditory system and the limbic system. This biological link makes it possible for sound to be processed almost immediately by the areas of the brain that are associated with long-term memory and the emotions. This link is also mediated at a subcortical level, making it possible for the processing of information despite higher cortical damage. This is evidenced clinically by the strong emotional responses to familiar music we observe in persons with memory deficits, such as multi-infarct dementia or Alzheimer's disease. Familiar songs become a tool for connecting to seemingly lost parts of the personality by providing a necessary link to the "self." (1999, p. 116)

Working from a neurological perspective using a behavioral model, Thaut (1999) writes about concepts he uses in applying music therapy to medical treatment. Focusing on clients who have suffered strokes and have resulting gait disorders, he uses rhythmic auditory stimulation (RAS) to "facilitate rehabilitation of movements that are intrinsically biologically rhythmical" (p. 239). He specifically uses music as a way of helping clients structure correct rhythmical elements of movement along with timing and anticipation. Studies have found that the length of the stride or step, the speed of walking, and the rhythm of walking have all shown improvement using rhythmic auditory stimulation (Hurt, Rice, McIntosh, & Thaut, 1998).

Humanistic Music Therapy

Humanistic music therapy focuses on helping clients achieve self-actualization and personal meaning. Humanistic music therapy can take place in a variety of settings such as medical hospitals, psychiatric hospitals, and schools. The focus is on recognizing the client as a complex being who exists in a relation to the world, and helping the client achieve meaning and fulfillment in a variety of life circumstances.

The clinical work of Nordoff and Robbins (1977) is an example of humanistic music therapy. In their early work, primarily with severely disabled children, they focused on what they term the "music child." They refer to this as follows:

> The entity in every child, which responds to musical experience, finds it meaningful and engaging, remembers music, and enjoys some form of musical expression. The Music Child is therefore the individualized musicality inborn in each child: The term has reference to the universality of musical sensitivity . . . it also points to the distinctly personal significance of each child's musical responsiveness. (1977, p. 1)

Therapists who train in this model of music therapy engage in rigorous training in developing musical resources. Therapists must become proficient in various scales and modes, atonality and bitonality, differentiating qualities of harmonic intervals, variety of tempi, dynamics, and rhythms. These musical resources support the Nordoff and Robbins technique known as "clinical improvisation." In this technique the therapist uses music as a way of creating a musical portrait of the child, thus providing him or her with a musical reflection of his or her existential life world. The therapist uses not only visual cues from the client, such as rocking or other behaviors, but also the therapist's own intuition and felt sense of the child in creating the improvisation. Once a connection is made in the music, the therapist works through the music to enhance that connection and bring the child into a musical relationship.

PRINCIPLES IN PRACTICE

This section examines several clinical examples of the practice of music therapy with a variety of populations and from a variety of approaches.

Music Therapy with Premature Infants

Jayne Standley (2000, 2003), a music therapy clinician/researcher in
the behavioral model of music therapy, has worked with and studied
premature infants in an NICU (neonatal intensive care unit). Since *in
utero* development has been interrupted for these infants, normal newborn development is often negatively impacted. An example of this is
the infant's ability to suck. Third-trimester fetuses *in utero* have been
observed engaging in nonnutritive sucking. Indeed, a newborn's sucking ability "is a critical behavior for both survival and neurological development" (Standley, 2000, p. 58). Standley cites a previous study
that indicates that sucking is a rhythmic behavior and that it "contributes to neurological development by facilitating internally regulated
rhythms" (Standley, 2000, p. 58). Yet, due to premature birth, these
infants frequently have difficulty sucking, resulting in loss of weight
and longer hospital stays.

Working as part of a team with a specialist in premature infant development, Standley developed a music therapy device to assist the infants in enhancing their sucking behavior. She created a pacifier that was
adapted to be pressure-sensitive. When activated by the infants' sucking,
it turned on a cassette tape player that played commercially recorded lul-
labies.

In a study conducted in 2000, Standley designed a 14-minute research protocol that included 2 minutes of silence followed by 5 minutes
of music contingent upon the infants sucking, another 2 minutes of silence, then another 5 minutes of music contingent upon the infants sucking. Using this receptive method of music therapy she found that the infants' sucking rates consistently increased during the music.

Stewart and Schneider (2000) approach the NICU from a humanistic perspective using improvisational music with the goal of impacting
the sound environment of this setting. Basing their work on indications
from the American Academy of Pediatrics that noise may be harmful to
newborns and fetuses, they first conducted a survey with staff regarding
their awareness of noise in the NICU. The results from this survey indicated that the staff perceived the NICU environment as being very noisy
and that the effect of this on the staff as well as the babies was indeed a
negative one. Their responses corroborate research that indicates that
noise in the environment can negatively affect the physiological stability
and sleep patterns of the infant (p. 90).

After the survey was conducted, the music therapist spent a 5-week period playing hammered dulcimer[1] in a central area of the NICU. The therapist used primarily improvised music, often matching the key of his music to the tone of the various medical machines that beep and chime, thus integrating environmental sounds into the music rather than adding music as a competing stimuli in the already noisy environment. The improvisations were usually either lullaby-like or classically inspired and were played with a direct intention on the part of the therapist to impact the atmosphere.

> As I play, I often imagine reaching out to the babies, playing for them in particular, keeping soothing and softening in mind. I play for the staff, too, since the music travels to all parts of the unit. . . . In the NICU I attempt to capture the sound and music needs of the moment, and to enter in it to give it a new shape and meaning so that it might be easier for the babies and the people on the unit to soften, to relax, to nurse, and to heal. (Stewart & Schneider, 2000, pp. 98–99)

After the 5-week intervention, the researcher interviewed the 25 staff members and found that for 24 of them the inclusion of music therapy in the NICU had been perceived as beneficial. "Staff experienced a reduced level of noise perception, a decreased level of tension and stress, a heightened consciousness of how they related to one another, and an overall 'lifting' of their mood" (p. 91).

Music Therapy and Developmental Delays

As discussed earlier, Boxill (1985) worked for many years with adults and children with developmental delays at a developmental center in New York City. One of her clients was Margarita, a 13½-year-old girl who had severe developmental delays. She exhibited no communicative speech, was preoccupied with inanimate objects, had autistic-like characteristics, and manifested self-stimulating and self-abusive behavior.

Boxill's initial approach to Margarita was to provide her with a reflection, in words and music, of her presence in the world. As Boxill states: "In initial encounters with a person who is unaware of self and others, mirrorring and matching what the person is doing or *not* doing in song, rhythmic chants, instrumental improvisations, and movement signify acceptance of that person" (p. 77).

---

[1]The hammered dulcimer is a box-like, wooden, stringed instrument played with small wooden mallets. The sound produced is delicate and bell-like.

Margarita received half-hour sessions twice weekly. In the first several weeks of treatment there was no overt response, but Boxill continued to sing familiar songs, making adaptations in the lyrics, and to improvise both instrumentally and vocally to constantly reflect Margarita's presence. In a session in Week 3 of treatment Boxill sang quietly in Margarita's ear while she played the autoharp and Margarita responded immediately by grabbing the autoharp, strumming the strings, and then placing her head near the strings. Boxill mirrored this behavior and it soon became a game during which Margarita smiled. Boxill then began improvising a song identifying what Margarita was doing. "Margarita, Margarita, Margarita is playing the harp, Margarita and Edi are playing the harp" (p. 79). Boxill reported that Margarita's body relaxed and she began to smile.

In a later session Margarita suddenly emitted a high-pitched sound to which Boxill provided a harmonic structure both vocally and on the piano and followed Margarita's tempo and dynamics. Margarita and Boxill exploded in laughter, enjoying their new level of contact.

Boxill developed the music theme that emerged from Week 3 into what she referred to as "the contact song." The contact song is defined as the "first two-way musical communication, the first overt musical indication initiated by the client of an awareness of the existence of another" (p. 80). In a later session, as Boxill played the contact song "Margarita" on the piano, Margarita came to the piano, sat on Boxill's lap, and played clusters of keys with her hand following the tonic-dominant harmonic progression of the song.

Boxill continued to develop the continuum of awareness, as discussed earlier, with Margarita. Through many experiences of improvising on the theme of the contact song at the piano, Margarita began to move from vocalizing to purposeful verbalizing, and eventually requesting to play the piano.

Music Therapy in Palliative Care

Colin Lee's seminal book *Music at the Edge: Music Therapy Experiences of a Musician with AIDS* (1996) provides a detailed and moving case study of Lee's work with Francis, a man with a diagnosis of AIDS. At the time Colin was working in England at the London Lighthouse, a residential center for people with HIV and AIDS. Francis received weekly hour-long sessions in the music therapy room at the hospital over the course of several months. The book includes a compact disk that allows the reader to hear as well as read about the process of therapy as it unfolded.

At the beginning of treatment, Francis is quite articulate and musical. While it is by no means a requirement for clients in music therapy to have musical training, occasionally one will encounter such a client. Lee's work revolves around the use of improvisation in music therapy. Francis and Lee at times improvise together, four hands at the keyboard, with Francis in the treble and Lee in the bass. At other times Francis improvises alone while Lee serves as a witness to the exploration. On some occasions Francis does verbally explore or process his improvisations, but on other occasions the experience of music stands on its own. For Francis the music experience is one of bringing his full being into the musical exploration, so much so that it serves as transformative experience, without the necessity of discussion. In Francis's words,

> . . . I feel this is almost like a testament. It's the only expression I have of a spiritual journey. The only time that I feel that I am living and communicating. The only moment that I feel I'm living the time I have left is when I am improvising. . . . When I'm doing these sessions with you I am actually living a moment: I'm actually living with somebody and producing something and revealing myself. When I'm improvising, when we are improvising together, I feel that I am saying something and living—and it's terribly important to me. (p. 78)

As the treatment progresses, we continue to hear in Francis own words how he is using the music and he offers his own interpretations. Referring to an improvisation, he states: "It was so full of life somehow, looking toward life rather than the more introvert expression of the first improvisation that I felt was more about possible loss and endings. Perhaps one complemented the other" (p. 43).

In the ensuing months of sessions, Lee and Francis explore a multitude of themes in music, many that revolved around the discrepancy between Francis's internal life and his external existence. After an improvisation Francis states:

> I think it is partly a striving to express one's own inner sense of harmony and beauty. This expression also reflects the knocks, destruction and pain that destroy the very basic life-giving feeling of expansion, the ability to feel what's going on around one. Is there an inner harmony that one strives for? Can one get into harmony without reality? Is that sometimes part of the journey? (p. 116)

Lee's response to Francis's self-revelatory soliloquy is "his music had accompanied him to this philosophical, ultimately theosophical, contemplation of the broader issues of life. It is unnecessary and inappropriate to attempt an interpretation of these words. They exist as a testament to the depth of his journey" (p. 116).

In later sessions, Francis, whose health was beginning to decline, continued to summon up his strength for these weekly improvisations. The music-making experience continued to be essential for Francis. While listening to the compact disk extracts of the sessions, a listener cannot help but be moved by the intensity of Francis's reality as brought to bear in these improvisations. In particular the final extract is especially striking. After improvising for some 45 minutes, Francis pauses. The pause is then followed by a series of repeated G's in octaves. They begin quite heavy and loud and over several minutes gradually diminish to a single note. This single note is repeated, becoming slower and fainter until it dies away, leaving only silence. While neither Lee nor Francis knew this would be their final session, it is clear from the music that this is a man on the very edge between life and death. It is a beautiful and agonizing improvisation that captures the finality of death in a way that simply cannot be put into words. These are Francis's words after what would be his final improvisation:

> Yes. . . . It's so magical. . . . I sit down and play that. It really puts other things into perspective. . . . It revises my sense of values and feelings. It makes me more secure in my leave of life. It reminds me of an ability of the soul. . . . Thank you for being there. I would like to name this improvisation "For Colin." (p. 139)

Within days, Francis had deteriorated and was no longer able to come to the hall for sessions. Although they played no more music together, Lee visited Francis several times prior to his death.

Music Therapy with a Geriatric Client with Advanced Alzheimer's Disease[2]

In a previous publication (Forinash & McKnight, 1999), a colleague and I documented doing clinical music therapy with Rose, a 90-year-old Jew-

---

[2]Parts of this section are excerpted from Forinash and McKnight (1999). Copyright 1999 by Barcelona Publishers. Adapted by permission.

ish immigrant and resident of a nursing home. Rose was blind, and also had chronic schizophrenia and Alzheimer's dementia. Her history was not clearly documented. It appeared that she had spent some years living in the woods in Poland to escape Nazi persecution. Some reports indicated that she may have lost a husband and a child during this time. She arrived in America, perhaps as a mail order bride, although records indicate that if she had married it had been a brief marriage.

Rose lived on the streets for much of her life in the United States. She frequently exhibited bizarre behaviors and was consequently placed in a psychiatric hospital, stabilized on medication, then discharged—which meant she returned to the streets. Once back on the street she would often stop taking her medication, thus continuing the cycle of hospitalizations. A woman who frequently passed Rose on the street was moved by her dilemma and decided to become her legal guardian. Rose, then in her 70s and suffering from advanced Alzheimer's disease, was admitted to a nursing home. Sally McKnight and I provided music therapy services to Rose at different times over a period of 5 years.

I first remember seeing Rose in other group settings where she would sit in her wheelchair, which had a laptop table attached, and pat the table as if she were smoothing laundry. Totally blind and having no communicative language (even when spoken to in Polish and when her expressions were translated into Polish), she seemed oblivious to her surroundings. Upon taking her out of a stimulating environment to a quiet area for an assessment, I was initially surprised by her level of musical relatedness. When I sang what I assumed would be familiar Yiddish and Hebrew songs, she responded by singing the final word in a phrase or humming along on pitch and in rhythm with me.

Based on her strong response, I chose to see Rose in both individual and group music therapy at the nursing home. In group, I placed her with three or four other clients who also demonstrated some ability to relate in the music, yet had severe physical limitations and some form of dementia. The goal was to help establish some sense of relatedness between them and to provide opportunities for self-expression and on occasion reminiscence. In individual sessions the focus remained the same; during assessment it had been clear that on some occasions the group experience could be too overwhelming and confusing and therefore would not enable her to relate and express.

When agitated, Rose would beat the laptop table attached to her chair with her hands. Given that she had bruised her hands on several occasions, a variety of mats were made to cover the table and protect her hands. When calmer, she would simply sit and gaze outward as if seeing a faraway place.

Over the 5-year period of treatment Rose's physical health failed. She became more impaired and underwent a partial leg amputation due to circulatory problems. Throughout this time her musical responsiveness remained stronger than I would have guessed was possible. Sally and I never felt we were providing maintenance treatment for Rose. Instead, we believed that through the musical relationship, we were providing her with a pathway of connection to humanity.

In 1998, I saw Rose for a series of four sessions that were videotaped. Sally McKnight and I independently analyzed these sessions. Our goal was to describe what occurred in the sessions, including Rose's participation and how the music was used, and to create a "narrative" on Rose's behalf of what her experience of the session might have been. It can be challenging to work with clients who are nonverbal. Use of a construct narrative, borrowed from qualitative research models (Aigen, 1997) allows us to attempt to illuminate a client's experience. The narrative we created for Rose is in *italics* in the following text.

Session 1

Rose sits in her elaborate wheelchair. Her white hair is neatly tied in a bun and she is dressed in a flowered housedress. She sits and pats her tray table.

[Pat, pat, pat, pat, pat.] *I have work to do. I must build up my work. I must keep busy. This work is familiar and I feel safe here, busy like this. I know what I need to do.* [Pat, pat, pat, pat, pat, pat.] *If I stop, the noise in my head gets too loud. Keeping busy helps stop the noise.* [Pat, pat, pat, pat.] *I hear something.* [Pause] *Is someone talking?* [Pause] *Is someone talking to me?* [Pause] *Is she talking to me? She is talking to me.*

I (as therapist) touch Rose's hand. She immediately sits back and stops patting. I hold her hand and say slowly, "Good morning, Rose. Good morning. Good morning." Rose replies, "Good morning?" I repeat, "Good morning. It is time for music." Rose withdraws her hand and continues her patting.

I am sitting close at her side and begin to sing a verse of Jimmy Davis and Charles Mitchell's "You Are My Sunshine," alternating using words and singing on "la." I pause at the cadence of the verse, waiting for Rose to join. Rose continues to pat. I sing it a second time, again pausing to create a space for Rose to join. Rose sings "la" in pitch on the final note of the song.

I hear her singing. I am so busy. I must finish my work. I hear her singing. It isn't that I really want to sing with her now; it is that I can't help but sing with her.

There is a pause in which Rose continues to pat. I start to strum the guitar and hum another Yiddish song. Rose is immediately still and listens for several seconds. I continue to sing on "la," pausing at the end of phrases to create space. Rose does not sing but continues to pat.

There is that music again. Do I know this music? Oh yes, I know this music. I need to keep up with my work. It is important to keep up and not stop. Go all the way to the edge. I don't want to miss a section.

I continue with the song but begin to reflect Rose's patting tempo in the tempo of her strum. Rose immediately stops patting and sits back, breathing deeply. When she does resume her patting, it is slower and has accents that reflect the phrasing in the music. We play together in this way for nearly a minute. As the song draws to a close, Rose slows her patting and stops just shy of the final cadence of the song. She rests for a few minutes and then resumes patting.

Oy, finally someone to help. She is helping me do my work. I need someone to help me with this. At least now I can take a short break. It is so much easier to work together. I am tired. [Pause] Back to work.

I begin singing another song and Rose is still, appearing to listen. Then her patting resumes. At the chorus I invite Rose to sing. She begins to sing, and does so in tempo and on pitch. She sings intermittently throughout four repetitions of the song. In the middle, I praise Rose's singing voice in both English and broken Yiddish. Rose continues to sing consistently throughout the final repetition of the song.

The music is so familiar. I know this music. It is my favorite. It is so beautiful. I love to sing it. What is she saying? She hears my singing.

[Pause] *She thinks my singing is beautiful! I love to sing this. She can hear me, ya!*

The song ends and I again praise Rose's singing and stroke her arm. Rose continues to pat. I rest my arm on the tabletop and Rose inadvertently pats my hand. She realizes she is touching someone and again becomes quiet. I leave my hand under hers and place my other hand on top of hers. Rose is quiet for nearly a minute.

That was beautiful music, but I must go back to work now. What's this? What am I touching? She is so close. She is touching me. That feels nice; she is helping me again. [Long pause] *But I have to keep going.*

Session 3

In this session Rose exhibits no patting behavior. She occasionally strokes the table and at times holds her hands, which are shaking strongly, out in front of her. As I sing a hello to Rose, she sings with me while her clasped hands shake. Rose completes several musical phrases by singing "la" on pitch and in tempo, then continues by adding several notes leading up to the ends of the musical phrases.

Sometimes it is hard to keep still. But today I am resting. When I am still, I can hear the music better. My hands don't want to stay still sometimes. I hear the music. It feels good to listen and to sing.

As the song ends, I reach out and stroke Rose's shoulder and say, "Your singing is so beautiful! Yeah?" Rose replies, "Yeah!" I then ask what she would like to sing and say, "How about 'Die Greene Koseene' (by Abe Schwartz and Chaim Prizant) Rose replies, "Ya, 'Die Greene Koseene' " and chuckles.

It feels good to sing. She hears me and she likes my singing. I am not alone in this. I hear the music. I feel it too. It makes me want to move. I want to sing that.

Later in the session I ask, "Shall we do 'Oif'n Pripetshik'?" (by Mark Warshavsky). Rose is quiet and I ask a second time. Rose chuckles and repeats the title of the song. She sings throughout this song using "la" rather than the lyrics. She sings in long, expressive phrases and needs little encouragement to continue. She seems very engaged and connected to the music. She has extended moments of music connection. Her voice is full and expressive. At times, she carries the melody while I simply accompany her on the guitar. She seems very involved in the music.

> *There is not so much noise in my head today. I can really hear the music. She waits for me and I join her singing. It is very beautiful. I feel so peaceful right now. It feels good to sing. I want to sing more. I will sing more. The music calls me in. I feel very warm now.*

At the end of the song, Rose seems tired and rests her head on her arm. I ask if she is getting tired and she replies, "Yes." I then end the session by singing a Yiddish lullaby while Rose listens.

In our viewing of the videotapes, we noticed several things. Rose turns toward the music throughout the sessions. When Rose is engaged in patting, it is often rhythmically synchronized to the music and reflects the musical phrasing as well. She seems to respond to the accents, dynamics, strum patterns, and articulations of the music by the quality of and patterns of her patting. At times it seems that her hands are almost "dancing" to the music.

There is a level at which Rose seems very aware. It is not a conscious awareness, but rather that she seems very aware of and sensitive to her environment and the atmosphere of her surroundings. There were many times when she seemed to respond to the mood and emotional expressions I made. One example of this is when I was genuinely moved by Rose's singing and praised her beautiful voice. Rose seems to understand the nature of the interaction and giggles, as one often does after receiving a compliment.

Rose received music therapy up until her death in 1999. In her work with Rose in previous music therapy groups, Sally recalled that even when Rose was not responding by singing, it was evident that she was aware of the music and would respond to changes in the sound. When she played her flute in a session for the first time, after having sung songs to keyboard or autoharp accompaniment, Rose would literally "sit up and take notice" and would stop her patting behavior when focusing on the music.

CONCLUSION

Music therapy continues to be a growing and developing field. It is expected that continuing research on the brain will yield results that will impact the practice of music therapy. Along with this development, there is no doubt of the ongoing need for humans to understand themselves in relation to the context in which they live. Music therapy and the other arts therapies will continue to address the biological as well as the emotional issues humans encounter.

REFERENCES

Aigen, K. (1997). *Here we are in music: One year with an adolescent music therapy group.* St. Louis, MO: MMB Music.

Boxill, E. H. (1985). *Music therapy for the developmentally disabled.* St. Louis, MO: MMB Music.

Bruscia, K. (1998). *Defining music therapy.* Gilsum, NH: Barcelona.

Davis, W. B., Gfeller, K. E, & Thaut, M. H. (1999). *An introduction to music therapy: Theory and practice* (2nd ed.). Boston: McGraw-Hill.

Dileo, C. (Ed.). (1999). *Music therapy and medicine: Theoretical and clinical applications.* Silver Spring, MD: American Music Therapy Association.

Forinash, M., & McKnight, S. (1999). Rose. In J. Hibben (Ed.), *Inside music therapy: Client experiences* (pp. 191–198). Gilsum, NH: Barcelona.

Grocke, D. (2002). *Opening remarks.* 10th World Congress of Music Therapy. Oxford, United Kingdom.

Hurt, C. P., Rice, R. R., McIntosh, G. C., & Thaut, M. H. (1998). Rhythmic auditory stimulation in gait training for patients with traumatic brain injury. *Journal of Music Therapy, 25,* 228–241.

Lee, C. (1996). *Music at the edge: Music therapy experiences of a musician with AIDS.* London & New York: Routledge.

Madsen, C. K. (1981). *Music therapy: A behavioral guide for the mentally retarded.* Lawrence, KS: National Association for Music Therapy, Inc.

Nordoff, P. & Robbins, C. (1977). *Creative music therapy.* New York: John Day.

Ruud, E. (1980). *Music therapy and its relationship to current treatment theories.* St. Louis, MO: MMB Music.

Scheiby, B. B. (1999). Music as symbolic expression: Analytical music therapy. In D. J. Weiner (Ed.), *Beyond talk therapy: Using movement and expressive techniques in clinical practice* (pp. 261–273). Washington, DC: American Psychological Association.

Standley, J. M. (2000). The effect of contingent music to increase non-nutritive sucking of premature infants. In J. V. Loewy (Ed.), *Music therapy in the neonatal intensive care unit* (pp. 57–70). St. Louis, MO: MMB Music.

Standley, J. M. (2003). *Music therapy with premature infants: Research and developmental interventions*. Silver Spring, MD: American Music Therapy Association.

Stewart, K., & Schneider, S. (2000). The effects of music therapy on the sound environment in the NICU: A pilot study. In J. V. Loewy (Ed.), *Music therapy in the neonatal intensive care unit* (pp. 85–100). St. Louis, MO: MMB Music.

Thaut, M. H. (1999). Music therapy in neurological rehabilitation. In W. B. Davis, K. E. Gfeller, & M. H. Thaut (Eds.), *An introduction to music therapy: Theory and practice* (2nd ed., pp. 221–247). New York: McGraw Hill.

Tomaino, C. M. (1998). *Clinical applications of music in neurologic rehabilitation*. St. Louis, MO: MMB Music.

Wheeler, B. (1983). A psychotherapeutic classification of music therapy practices: A continuum of procedures. *Music Therapy Perspectives, 1,* 8–12.

Winnicott, D. (1971). *Playing and reality.* New York: Routledge.

Wolberg, L. R. (1977). *The techniques of psychotherapy* (3rd ed.). New York: Grune & Stratton.

Dance/Movement Therapy

SUSAN T. LOMAN

The love of dance and the desire to help others are combined in the field of dance/movement therapy. According to the American Dance Therapy Association (ADTA), dance/movement therapy is defined as "the psychotherapeutic use of movement as a process which furthers the emotional, cognitive, physical and social integration of the individual" (available at *www.adta.org*). Dance/movement therapists work with people of all ages with a wide range of mental and physical abilities. They work with both individuals and groups. Their primary goals include removing the obstacles people have in expressing themselves, relating to others, or accepting their bodies or selves. With clients who report that they "hide behind words" or cannot find the words to express themselves in traditional verbal therapy, "movement doesn't lie" and dance/movement therapy can facilitate the embodiment and identification of problems leading to insight and lifestyle changes. It is a creative and action-oriented process that encourages new behaviors and symbolically communicates hidden emotions, releases anxiety, and serves as a vehicle to integrate body, mind, and spirit.

Dance/movement therapists have had success in engaging children with autism as well as individuals with eating disorders and body image issues. Dance/movement therapies are effective with infants who cannot communicate through words, but are extremely expressive in their use of movement and sounds. Since dance/movement therapies intervene on a nonverbal level, it is a modality appropriate for people who have difficulties that began preverbally or with those who have suffered bodily trauma such as accidents, illness, physical or sexual abuse, or posttraumatic stress disorder. As Lewis (1996) describes:

> Reclaiming preverbal memories which lie in the body and bodily sensations allow both the client and therapist to reconstruct early trauma. Winnicott has stated that many memories are "pre-verbal, non verbal and unverbalizable" (1971, p. 130). Since many memories of abuse occur prior to language, they are often held in unconscious somatic schemata that can only be recalled by kinesthetic and movement reconstruction. (p. 101)

HISTORY

Rooted in the use of dance throughout early human history for healing, dance/movement therapy officially became a profession in the 1960s. Pioneers in dance/movement therapy drew from their backgrounds in modern dance as an effective vehicle for the expression of emotions, authenticity, spontaneity, and community. They also capitalized on the cultural basis for dance and movement, realizing that traditionally dance was used in rituals to cure ills of all kinds. The universal language of dance transcends social, racial, gender, cultural, and environmental differences.

Founders of the field were guided by their experiences in teaching dance classes to those not necessarily interested in performing. Their students seemed to crave the enjoyment of using their bodies artistically and expressively. When Marian Chace, a Denishawn dancer in the 1930s, opened a studio and began teaching, she found that many of her students were not planning to become performers but were still motivated to attend class. Students who began the courses feeling depressed reported that their moods had lifted as a result of dancing. Chace's skill as a dance teacher became more widely known, and in 1942 she was invited to bring dance to psychiatric patients at St. Elizabeths Hospital in Washington, DC. She had tremendous success using dance to foster communication, establish empathy, and promote social interaction with hospitalized patients who were receiving minimal treatment.

When Chace was working in hospitals, antipsychotic medication was not yet available and patients often moved with gestures that were considered bizarre and abnormal. Chace met these patients on their own terms, wheeling her record player onto the psychiatric ward. Soon a group of people would gather. She began moving with patients to their own rhythms and in their often nonverbal worlds, gradually gaining their trust. Eventually Chace was able to reach even the most isolated patients through dance and movement. Other pioneers on the West Coast had similar experiences combining dance and various forms of psychotherapy. Mary Whitehouse (1986) developed a practice called "Authentic Movement" which integrated Carl Jung's concept of "active imagination." Arising from an inner awareness Authentic Movement involves a process of moving from the inside out, often with eyes closed, to bring buried information about the self to consciousness.

Dosamantes-Beaudry (1997) provides some historical insights on the field's evolution:

> First generation dance therapy pioneers (e.g., Marian Chace, Blanche Evan, Liljan Espenak, Mary Whitehouse, Trudi Schoop and Alma Hawkins) intuitively understood the value of embodied experience in altering human consciousness. They recognized that the creative and healing elements of dance could be made available to ordinary people as well as to people institutionalized with emotional disorders.
>
> . . . A major achievement of second generation dance therapists was the creation of an expanded vision of DMT [dance/movement therapy] which included psychodynamic concepts borrowed from Psychoanalytic and Jungian Schools of Psychology. Such concepts as an interpersonal view of human development, an understanding of unconscious processes and the workings of transference and countertransference reactions within the context of the therapeutic relationship were all introduced into the mainstream vocabulary of dance therapists by several second generation dance therapists with exposure or training in these psychologies. (pp. 17–19)

THEORETICAL ORIENTATIONS

The field of dance/movement therapy is based on the belief that healthy functioning depends on the integration of the mind, the body, and the spirit. When there is a lack of such integration, an individual, group, or family may suffer from a variety of psychophysical disorders. Dance/movement therapy is a form of psychotherapy that utilizes movement as the medium of interaction and intervention promoting change. The following section summarizes the major theoretical orientations within the field of dance/movement therapy.

Chace Approach

A basic tool for establishing nonverbal relationships used by dance/movement therapists is called *mirroring*, or *attunement*. Marian Chace, a major pioneer in the field reflected, through her own muscular activity, the body movement of her patients. She was able to meet her patients where they were emotionally on a nonverbal, movement level of communication.

Marian Chace's core concepts of working in groups, utilizing rhythmic body action, and communicating through dance and movement are considered fundamental (see Figure 4.1). She states:

> Dance therapy is the specific use of rhythmic bodily action employed as a tool in the rehabilitation of patients. . . . The dance therapist combines verbal and non-verbal communication to enable a patient to express feeling, to participate in human relationships, to increase personal self-esteem, to develop a more realistic concept of his body image, and

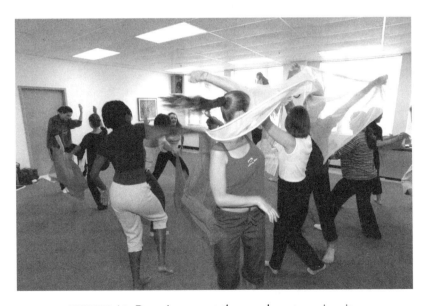

FIGURE 4.1. Dance/movement therapy class at a university.

through all these to achieve some feeling of relaxation and enjoyment. (1993, p. 247)

The main method in initiating trusting and meaningful contact with patients is mirroring, or joining them in movement. Levy (1992) describes this concept that Marian Chace developed as a way of "reflecting a deep emotional acceptance and communication" (p. 25). According to Levy, the therapist takes the individual's nonverbal and verbal communications seriously and assists him or her in broadening, expanding, and clarifying them. In other words, Chace believed that through recognizing the person on a deep and genuine level, the person was validated and his or her emotional experience was accepted. Susan Sandel (1993a), a former student of Chace, expands on the concept of "mirroring" using the term "empathic reflection," stating that it is

> the dance therapist's mode for developing multiple empathic connections between him/herself and the clients, and one means by which the therapist structures a nonjudgmental, supportive environment which is conducive to sharing and growth. The therapist utilizes both verbal and nonverbal cues from the participants in assessing the prevailing moods, affects, and concerns; this information guides the way in which the therapist develops the flow of movement interaction as it unfolds during the session. Empathic reflection is both a means of acquiring information and a method of intervening in dance therapy. (p. 98)

Judith Kestenberg calls movement empathy "attunement," observing that it involves harmony between movers. Regarding "complete attunement" in the mother–infant interaction, Kestenberg (1975) notes that complete attunement consists of mutual empathy and that "there is not only a sameness of needs and responses, but also a synchronization in rhythms" (p. 161). The experience of attunement requires a process of kinesthetic identification. Muscular tensions felt in one person are also felt in the other. It is not necessary to duplicate the shape of the movement. Visual or touch attunement with a child or adult who is upset can lead to soothing. The degree of tension exhibited by the child or adult can be initially matched and then developed into less intense, more soothing patterns (Loman, 1998).

Many first-generation dance/movement therapists apprenticed with Chace. Current students of dance/movement therapy continue to study Chace's approach, and her methods are still practiced widely (Chaiklin & Schmais, 1993; Levy, 1995; Sandel, 1993a; Stanton-Jones, 1992).

Integrated Developmental Approach

Another widely used approach in the field is developmental dance/ movement therapy. Dance/movement therapists observe developmental phases in movement and help clients work through developmental blocks, regressions, and delays (Lewis, 1986, 2002; Loman, 1998; Loman & Merman, 1996; Naess, 1982; Sandel, 1993b; Siegel, 1984).

An integrated developmental approach draws from psychodynamic, ego psychological, Jungian, and relational models. The approach encompasses a solid movement and body-level understanding of the individual, interpersonal relationships, groups, and family systems throughout the life cycle. The framework for understanding human development, based primarily on Erik Erikson, Anna Freud, Judith Kestenberg, Jean Baker Miller and colleagues, Margaret Mahler, and Donald Winnicott, fosters awareness of the significant life challenges encountered at each stage of the life cycle. Each stage can be approached from a body–mind–spirit perspective.

Object relations theories, particularly those outlined by Mahler, Pine, and Bergman (1975) and Winnicott (1965), with their body-movement foundations, provide an understanding of the phases of separation/ individuation and the nature of interpersonal relationships. The "relational model" developed by Jean Baker Miller and colleagues (Jordan, Kaplan, Miller, Stiver, & Surrey, 1991) offers concepts about the ongoing nature of relationships that can thrive throughout an individual's development when there is mutual empowerment, trust, and empathy. A developmental dance/movement orientation addresses an individual's intrapsychic, interpersonal, and spiritual evolution.

Authentic Movement Approach

Many dance/movement therapists incorporate the practice of "authentic movement" in their work. Authentic movement was first developed by dance therapist Mary Whitehouse (1986).

Dance/movement therapist Joan Chodorow (1986) describes the process:

> Dance/movement is one of the most direct ways to reach back to our earliest experiences. Movers frequently lie on or move close to the ground. By attending to the world of bodily felt sensations, the mover recreates a situation that is in many ways similar to that of an infant who swims in a sensory-motor world. The presence of the analyst/witness enables re-

enactment and re-integration of the earliest preverbal relationship(s). It is here that images of the transference and the countertransference may be most clearly recognized. (pp. 97–98)

Janet Adler (1996, 2003), a student of Mary Whitehouse, has spent many years teaching, refining, and practicing authentic movement. She observes that this method is grounded in the relationship between a mover and a witness and that

> the heart of the practice is about the longing, as well as the fear, to see ourselves clearly. The mover, who is the expert on his own experience, works with eyes closed in the presence of the witness, who sits still to the side of the movement space. The mover listens inwardly for the occurrence of impulse toward movement. This movement, visible or invisible to the witness, shapes the mover's body as it becomes a vessel through which unconscious material awakens into consciousness. As he internalizes his witness's desire to accept him, to accept his suffering as well as his beauty, embodiment of the density of his personal history empties, enabling him at times to feel seen by the witness, and more importantly to see himself clearly. . . . (1996, pp. 85–86)

The person who witnesses the movement essentially internalizes the movements and attends to personal experiences of judgment, interpretation, and projection in response to what he or she sees. Many practitioners of dance/movement therapy use this approach in their clinical work. In summary, the concepts inherent to authentic movement such as inner listening and witnessing others and the self are believed to be transformative in and of themselves (Musicant, 2001).

ASSESSMENT IN DANCE/MOVEMENT THERAPY

The ability to analyze and interpret nonverbal behavior and assess the individual's body attitude and psychophysical characteristics is essential in dance/movement therapy. The observations guide the therapist in developing an accurate assessment and a coherent treatment plan. Dance/movement therapists have been quite successful in their ability to establish relationships with clients, to empathize, and to provide a vehicle for transformation and healing through the use of the body. The therapeutic process, however, may appear mysterious to those not trained in dance/movement therapy. The language and psychological implications of body movement are difficult to describe clearly and communicate to other professionals. To bridge this gap, a comprehensive system of movement analysis, using its own vocabulary, is of great value.

Feder and Feder (1998) summarize major assessment tools in dance/ movement therapy that have been used to describe movement and to evaluate outcome in dance/movement therapy as follows:

- *Laban movement analysis (LMA), or effort/shape analysis.* The LMA is based on the work of Rudolf Laban and has been modified by his students and colleagues. The LMA has been the foundation for other notation systems and several checklists. It has been used in a variety of ways in personality assessment, such as the connection between personality traits and body movements. The LMA is a system and a vocabulary for describing qualitative aspects of movement, based on four interrelated components: body, effort, space, and shape. For example, on a *body* level, the therapist notes what body parts and actions are used to perform a given movement. In brief, *effort* is the qualitative changes in movement exertion, *space* is how individuals move their bodies within the environment, and *shape* refers to individuals' forms or shapes made with movement through space.
- *Kestenberg Movement Profile.* The Kestenberg Movement Profile is a system with roots in LMA that is used both to describe and to interpret body movement. Because it is so widely used by contemporary dance/movement therapists, an expanded description of its application is provided later in this section.
- *Espenak's (1981) movement diagnostic tests.* These tests have been developed to identify personality using movement as a measure.
- *Differential diagnosis dance/movement assessments.* Examples include Davis's Movement Psychodiagnostic Inventory (Davis, Cruz, & Berger, 1995) and Kalish-Weiss's Body Movement Scale for Autistic and Other Atypical Children (BRIAAC; Kalish-Weiss, 1976).

Kestenberg Movement Profile

To give the reader a better idea of the use of assessment in dance/movement therapy, the Kestenberg Movement Profile (KMP) is described in more detail because it has been used by many therapists as the assessment tool of choice (Loman & Merman, 1996). This integrated system, bridging Laban movement analysis with object relations and psychodynamic theories, can be used as a developmental and psychological tool for diagnosis, treatment planning, and intervention for individuals of all ages (Kestenberg Amighi, Loman, Lewis, & Sossin, 1999). Some dance/movement therapists use the KMP as a survey of movement qualities to catalogue nonverbal behavior in typical as well as clinical populations.

The KMP is a movement-based profile, consisting of qualitative information in nine diagrams that display more than 100 different possible qualities of movement in an individual's movement repertoire. The KMP evaluates an individual's level of developmental functioning, movement preferences, and areas of psychological harmony and conflict. It is designed to observe natural movement processes and does not require the client to follow any specific instructions, allowing it to be used with any population, age group, or level of ability. When KMPs of two or more individuals are compared, interpersonal compatibility can be measured.

Once a KMP is completed, it serves as a movement portrait upon which to base a developmental assessment and a treatment plan. Knowing the framework of the KMP can help therapists become more aware of the strengths and limitations in the individual's movement vocabulary. KMP assessments reveal potential areas of vulnerability between people, such as a child and his or her parent, and areas of compatibility and incompatibility between them. KMP observations can be used to determine whether a child has reached an age-adequate developmental level. In both children and adults, it can show areas of regression and chances for developmental growth. Like other assessments, KMP findings can be utilized to develop ideas to enhance personal strengths, reduce stress, and support the individual. In work with families or groups, the KMP can help the therapist develop interventions to enhance communication among individuals.

In dance/movement therapy, the therapist works toward expanding the individual's movement repertoire to further develop coping skills and personal strengths. An important goal in dance/movement therapy is to increase the individual's movement repertoire, thus providing him or her with more options for dealing with interpersonal as well as intrapersonal experiences. After a period of dance/movement therapy treatment, another KMP assessment is often conducted to measure whether or not the interventions were effective and whether the individual's movement repertoire expanded.

Movement qualities studied in the KMP reflect individuals' styles of learning and cognition, expression of needs and feelings, modes of relating, styles of defense, and dynamics for coping with the environment. The psychodynamically oriented therapist can use the KMP to determine motivation, temperament, affects, learning styles, object relations, ego development, defense mechanisms, and coping skills. The KMP can be used to pursue varied research goals and can be used to pre- and posttest clients in dance/movement therapy to measure change over time.

DANCE/MOVEMENT THERAPY
PRINCIPLES IN PRACTICE

Dance/movement therapy is a modality that works particularly well with children because it uses body movements to assess nonverbal behavior and employs self-expression through movement as the treatment modality. The language of movement is already known and understood by most children. Through the language of the body, therapist and child can co-create moment-to-moment movement dialogues. The dance/movement therapist develops nonverbal relationships, intervenes through movement, and helps the child process any traumatic experiences. Providing a therapeutic relationship within a predictable and consistent therapeutic "container" helps promote trust between therapist and client.

Dance/movement therapy with children and adolescents is utilized within general and special education, in public and private schools, and in mental health settings (Kornblum, 2002). Infants and young children at risk can benefit from the inclusion of dance/movement therapy in early intervention programs. Parents and family members are included in the treatment to support and enhance the growth of the child and to improve the functioning of the family.

In work with adolescents, dance/movement therapy is helpful with identity and gender issues, body image problems, and eating disorders. It provides an experiential process through which teenagers can express themselves, discharge feelings in a creative and safe way, release tension, reduce stress, establish trust, and develop meaningful relationships.

Case Example: Group of Teenage Parents and Their Babies

Background

The following is a case example of a group of teen parents and their children in a high school setting. The purpose of the group was to encourage good communication skills between parent and child via dance/movement therapy. We (myself and a cotherapist) wanted to support the teens in the beginning stages of their new roles as parents and in their new relationships with their children. We also wanted to enhance their personal growth, self-expression, and confidence. By providing a base of support for the teens, we hoped to help them develop an awareness of their children and their uniqueness, individuality, and creativity.

In the early stages, the teen parents learned to understand nonverbal cues and movement development within a supportive environment. The therapists set boundaries and adjusted them as needed. The teenage parents attended the group with their children, played with them, and strengthened their relationship in a social environment designed to support self-esteem.

The teens were encouraged to play with their own and other teens' children and to participate in creative movement interactions. A feeling of community spirit was developed through mutual sharing of the children's new accomplishments. As dance/movement therapists, we emphasized nonverbal interaction and the predictable stages of development that could be observed and promoted in movement. Teaching the teens to attune to their children through nonverbal empathy (Chace, 1993; Kestenberg, 1975) helped them to recognize and understand their children's needs and temperaments and their level of development (see Figure 4.2).

For example, one young parent in particular was becoming very frustrated with her child's excessive crying bouts. I modeled a Chacian approach to her child in a typical way that dance/movement therapists use to relate with clients. I matched the child's crying rhythm in movement as well as in sound, thus communicating to the child an understanding of his feelings, rather than giving the message that it is not okay to feel upset. I did this by reproducing his muscle tension and release in my own body, as Chace (1993) describes. I used my breath to provide both support and comfort, with the intention of converting the child's crying into slower, calmer breathing rhythms (Kestenberg, 1975). As I held the child securely, breathed with him, and matched his tension patterns while dancing a modified waltz rhythm with him, he began to settle down. The mother was surprised, but pleased by the response. After seeing the positive results of my interaction, she tried this method herself. Later, she reported that she felt less frustrated now because she had a proactive approach to soothe his crying.

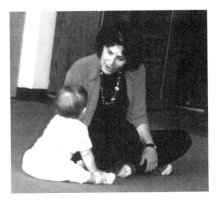

FIGURE 4.2. Dance/movement therapist, Susan Loman, establishing relationship with child through attunement to movements and sounds.

The therapist's responses of rhythm duplication via attunement on an embodied level helped lay the foundations for the development of a mutually empathic relationship. Through exceptionally simple, yet effective, interventions and responses, both child and therapist experienced a deepened level of connection reflecting being truly seen and understood.

Using a Nonverbal Approach

In our work with these teen parents and their children, we created a "holding environment" (Winnicott, 1965; Loman, 1994), a safe, supportive place where parents and children interact, share, and learn. The room was "child-proofed," so there were no objects with which the children could hurt themselves. There was a consistent structure to activities as well as consistency in leadership. The children could predict what the environment would look like and in what order activities would take place. We offered props such as soft balls and baskets, parachutes and scarves, tunnels, and songs to sing hellos and good-byes to impart a sense of fun.

The teens were encouraged to play with their own and other teens' children and to participate in all activities. The parents were also encouraged to share their observations of the children's new accomplishments as they rolled over, crawled, sat up, stood, walked, danced, and made sounds and words. Within this relaxed atmosphere, teens interacted and communicated with each other and the dance/movement therapists, also experiencing a "holding environment" similar to that of their children.

Results

During early sessions, the teens expressed very little feeling. Initially, they seemed to have an absence of curiosity, did not look at their babies, or did not smile frequently. When they did interact with the babies, they treated them like inanimate objects, tickling them, or pulling them up in postures they were not ready for. They sat with muted affect that was also observable in the babies' lack of animation and facial expression. Most parents were initially defensive or had a hostile attitude that made it hard to reach them easily.

Eventually, the teen parents became more comfortable with the predictable holding environment we provided and the consistent membership of the leaders, and they began to open up and connect more with each other, their babies, and the therapists. The pervading lack of feeling and expression was reduced. As a group, they became more attuned and responsive to their babies and initiated activities and conversations. Eventually, the teens became more empathetic in their responses to their own children and in the degree to which they were appropriately attached to their babies. One teen who had a problematic childhood herself and needed a lot of support and empathetic responsiveness finally began smiling more at her baby and holding her more often. Finally, the teens began to nurture each other's babies and responded warmly and enthusiastically to others' children.

Case Example: Individual Dance/Movement Therapy with an Adolescent

Sally, a 17-year-old girl who is developmentally delayed and has cerebral palsy, attends a school for developmentally delayed children and adolescents (Loman & Foley, 1996). She has limited speech but is able to understand language and to respond appropriately. She was referred to dance/movement therapy to work on the following goals: to improve communication skills, to decrease tactile defensiveness, to improve her ability to relax, to increase attention span and eye contact, and to redirect inappropriate behavior.

Sally was seen individually once a week for half-hour sessions over a period of 9 months. The sessions were held in a large all-purpose room that contained various equipment and props. During the first several sessions Sally was quite distracted, often giggling uncontrollably and unable to maintain eye contact. She could not stay with any interaction for very long. At times she ran around the room wanting the therapist to chase her. Other times she kicked her legs while lying on the mat as if having a temper tantrum.

The therapist's initial goals were to establish trust and to develop a relationship. As in all dance/movement therapy work, the therapist wanted to create a therapeutic container, or "holding environment." Creating consistency, predictability, and stability in the relationship paves the way for trust to flourish. Creativity, spontaneity and intense dynamics can then be contained within the consistent structure. The therapist incorporated the crucial KMP concepts of "attunement," based on a sharing of qualities of muscle tension, and "shape-flow adjustment," based on a similarity of breathing patterns and the shape of the body, the nonverbal counterparts to empathy and trust (Kestenberg, 1975). The KMP movement assessment informed the therapist about how Sally moved, expressed herself nonverbally, and at what level of development she was functioning. She seemed to focus better when she and the therapist moved together using simple patting rhythms typical of a young child using a "biting rhythm" around the age of teething. When the therapist began to give simple commands such as "Can we hold hands down the hall?," she began to respond.

Several weeks later Sally initiated a peek-a-boo game while hiding under a large cloth. Peek-a-boo involves turning and twisting movements, which were new movement qualities for Sally. While under the cloth, Sally and the therapist looked at each other and then looked away. This game seemed to put them in the "practicing stage of development" described by Mahler et al. (1975). A shift occurred when she began to push the therapist away by using the strain–release rhythm (Kestenberg Amighi et al., 1999), the next stage in the KMP developmental framework that is typical of an 18-month-old child. At first the therapist allowed her to have an effect on her bodily positioning and responded by collapsing down. Remembering that during the strain–release phase children like to test limits and boundaries, the therapist wondered if Sally might be testing her through this pushing movement, asking herself if the therapist was strong enough to contain her. The therapist changed her position and resisted being moved. At the end of the session the therapist told her it was time to go and Sally put on her shoes without resistance. Perhaps meeting her pushing energy with strength helped Sally feel more secure. While they walked back to Sally's classroom, Sally did not giggle as she usually did.

A dance/movement therapist drawing on a developmental approach can identify themes that pertain to specific phases of movement development. The therapist can support the client's exploration of these developmental themes within the safety of the therapeutic environment. When clients indicate, through changes in movement patterns, that they are ready to explore the next phase of development, the therapist will be ready to provide a suitable phase-appropriate holding environment. The therapist can alter the approach to the client in accordance with the client's needs. This is especially important when the client makes a transition to a more mature phase of development.

During the next few sessions Sally was able to relax more and to maintain eye contact longer. She appeared pleased to see the therapist and smiled openly when she asked her to come for the sessions.

In later sessions, interactions of "tug of war" and "keep-away" developed, continuing with the approach–avoidance theme that had begun in earlier sessions. At one point, the therapist pantomimed that she was looking for the rope, which Sally was holding. Sally laughed and hid the rope from the therapist. The relationship began to show signs of healthy spontaneity and playfulness. The therapist helped Sally express her intense feelings through the "tug of war" movement expression within the safety of the therapeutic container. The developmental approach helped guide Sally to channel her intense feelings into phase-specific, creative outlets.

As the sessions drew to a close, Sally made progress in maintaining eye contact, relaxing, making more sounds, cooperating, and staying focused for longer periods. The push–pull dynamics became subsumed into games such as mutual sit-ups where they would take turns pulling each other up from a lying-down position.

Developmental Sequencing

Through the therapist's conscious attunement with Sally's developmental rhythms, she enabled Sally to establish contact in a way that was not only safe and trust building, but also enticing. Their interactions highlighted Sally's willingness for further engagement, created in an environment of mutual exploration.

Her knowledge of the KMP developmental movement phases helped inform the therapist at which developmental stage Sally was functioning and which behaviors were expected for that stage. The therapist was better able to provide more specific ways of attuning in keeping with Sally's developmental level. During vulnerable transitional periods when Sally was entering a new phase of development, it was essential for the therapist to support Sally's practicing of the newly emerging movement patterns. The therapist helped facilitate Sally's working through of unresolved developmental issues.

Containment

Through observation and interaction, the therapist identified that Sally lacked certain indulgent movement patterns and showed an excess of "fighting movement" qualities. The therapist was able to channel Sally's fighting movement patterns by creating a container for the emotional expression. Since Sally was prone to disorganize readily and had poor communication skills, a developmentally based form of intervention provided the opportunity for Sally to express herself at her own level while developing more mature patterns. Over time she was able to improve her impulse control, coping skills, and social skills.

Group and Individual Case Examples: Dance/Movement Therapy with Adults

Dosamentes-Beaudry (1984) delineates distinctive characteristics that distinguish dance/movement therapy from traditional verbal psychotherapy:

> . . . (a) the greater weight given to clients' derivation of personal meaning from their nonverbal experiencing; using movement and imagery as media of experience and emotional expression, (b) the fact that the therapist consistently focuses and maintains the client's attention on his/her bodily-felt experiencing while the client assumes the dual role of experiencer and observer to her/his own experiential process (c) the therapist's acceptance of a somatopsychic view of a client's resistance which encompasses the experience of working through body blocks, blocks in the flow of body movement as well as breaks in the flow of the client's images and verbalized associations, and (d) the attention paid by the therapist to nonverbal aspects of the ongoing therapeutic relationship. (p. 152)

Dance/Movement Therapy with a Group of Adults on an Inpatient Unit

This dance/movement therapy group took place on an adult inpatient unit and included middle-aged and older adults (Loman & Merman,

1996). The predominant mood of this first dance/movement therapy group was depression and withdrawal demonstrated by the presence of deanimated affect and minimal eye contact, communication, and interpersonal relationships.

The group members sat in a circle on chairs while rhythmic, nonintrusive music played. At first the therapist sat quietly, feeling present with the patients. During this warm-up period, she invited them to sense their body's weight, to become aware of the support of the chairs behind their backs and under their seats, and to feel where their bodies felt comfortable or uncomfortable that day. She asked them to become aware of their breathing, and how they grew wider on the inhalation and narrower on the exhalation. She then asked the patients to rub their backs gently against the back of the chair and to try lifting and dropping an arm to the side. The warm-up helped them move from deanimation, reflecting feelings of depression, caution, and helplessness, to movement qualities expressive of calmness, patience, and adaptability.

The therapist recognized the early developmental issues of give-and-take as a current theme. She used the space, chairs, her voice, and simple directions to provide support and structure. As the group began to feel supported and accepted, they were able to get in touch with themselves on a body level.

Soothing rocking movements ensued, followed by rhythmic opening and closing of the hands in the same quality. Active patting and self-massaging of body parts helped to increase self-awareness and self-nurturance. More energetic tapping of hands and feet followed in a snapping type of rhythm (Kestenberg Amighi et al., 1999), serving heightened alertness, definition of body parts and boundaries, and differentiation. The group was able to synchronize while moving in rhythm. As individual mobility and group energy increased, patients began to become aware of each other, to look, to speak, and to interact. In the Chace approach therapists pick up on the group's rhythmic action and develop it. As Chaiklin and Schmais (1993) note, "As feelings are expressed in a shared rhythm, each member draws from the common pool of energy and exeriences a heightened sense of strength and security" (pp. 80–81).

Group members reached across the circle, out of their own personal space, to shake hands with others and to pat a neighbor's hand, shoulder, knee, or foot. Participants no longer relied solely on the therapist's suggestions but spontaneously offered their own. The group's mood changed from one of isolation and depression to one of hesitation followed by purposeful greeting, discovery, and sharing (Loman & Merman, 1996).

Individual Dance/Movement Therapy

This case example illustrates a developmental approach with an individual client seen in private practice over time (Loman & Merman, 1999). The client began dance/movement therapy to address her eating disorder and the loneliness and fatigue she experienced following the breakup of a relationship 5 years earlier. To help the therapist make an initial assessment, the therapist asked her to improvise. The client ran around the room in large circles using hurried movement. While her body demonstrated movement that was direct and focused, her head frequently moved around with flexibility. The differences in movement qualities in various body parts indicated a conflict. While talking, she encroached on the therapist's space as she used small continuous finger motions on her own body.

The therapist's impression of the client was that she was a motivated, goal-directed, but possibly driven woman who, while expending much energy, lacked an ability to recuperate. Her movements suggested conflicts and contrast between her ability to function independently and her expression of unmet developmental needs (her use of self-soothing rhythms, self-touch, and the inappropriate proximity she created).

As the course of treatment progressed, it became clear that this client preferred to use large movements through the space. During one session, the therapist suggested that she try to improvise staying in one place. Standing still, she shortened down with bent knees, her chest hollowing back in and her head drooping forward and down. Throughout her body there was a preponderance of low muscle tone, indicating deanimation. Limply and gradually she sank to the floor, ending in a small heap. When asked what she was feeling, she noted with surprise: "Depression."

During the verbal processing of this session, the conflicts expressed in her movement were discussed. Her use of fast-paced movement was connected to her fast-paced achievement-oriented lifestyle. Her use of acceleration while moving forward helped her run away from feelings of dependency, deprivation, and possible rage. The price she paid for not facing her feelings was exhaustion, loneliness, and depression. She related her movement patterns to her lifestyle and supported the current discovery of an inner feeling (which also helped her to feel when she is hungry and full) now that she was able to slow down. She reported that she felt seen and understood through the movement interactions and the verbal processing.

Therapy progressed from structured movement with the therapist to increasingly unstructured, improvised movement by the client on her own. Subsequent treatment dealt with working through issues of depression and rage relating to her unstable, often absent mother and her verbally and physically abusive father. She felt she repeatedly created patterns in relationships and jobs that led to eventual rejection. It took a period of time for her own angry feelings to surface and find tolerable expression through movement and words, and finally in relationship to the therapist. During the middle phase of treatment she would stomp the ground, expressing anger and frustration. Later, she was able to verbalize anger toward her parents and the therapist.

During the end of treatment, the woman punched forward and ran and leapt with strength or lightness, expressing exuberance as well as anger. Another observed sign of improvement was the increase in the number of "postural movements" or the use of the whole body (Kestenberg Amighi et al., 1999). More postural movement is considered an indication of increased emotional and physical involvement. Although the client's proclivity remained "being on the move," recuperative phases allowed her to rest, to take vacations, and begin a serious relationship. During the termination session, she sat calmly and comfortably at an appropriate distance from the therapist, spoke softly, and was able to share silence. Previously, this highly verbal client was prone to intellectualization, rationalization, and isolation. The movement work enabled her to access previously cut-off bodily and emotional feeling states and provided her with a way to express and integrate aspects of herself. She was then able to transform intrapersonal and relational issues through both movement and verbal modes of communication. The client's movement repertoire evolved over the course of treatment, building more mature, harmonious movement patterns and reflecting emotional growth and integration (Loman & Merman, 1999).

CONCLUSION

Dance/movement therapy helps individuals of all ages reconnect with their whole selves: body, mind, and spirit. When people lose touch with the body's expressiveness and have difficulty releasing feelings, stress, or tension, dance/movement therapy helps individuals to capitalize on strengths and imparts a sense of connectedness and joy in their lives through both short and long-term intervention. It is an action-oriented, creative, and spontaneous therapy leading to growth and change and facilitating people's natural ability to express themselves and communicate more fully through their own bodies.

REFERENCES

Adler, J. (1996). The collective body. *American Journal of Dance Therapy, 18*(2), 81–94.

Adler, J. (2003). American Dance Therapy Association 37th annual conference keynote address: From autism to the discipline of authentic movement. *American Journal of Dance Therapy, 25*(1), 5–16.

Chace, M. (1993). Dance alone is not enough. In S. Sandel, S. Chaiklin, & A. Lohn (Eds.), *Foundations of dance/movement therapy: The life and work of Marian Chace* (pp. 246–251). Columbia, MD: Marian Chace Memorial Fund of the American Dance Therapy Association.

Chaiklin, S., & Schmais, C. (1993). The Chace approach to dance therapy. In S. Sandel, S. Chaiklin, & A. Lohn (Eds.), *Foundations of dance/movement therapy: The life and work of Marian Chace* (pp. 75–97). Columbia, MD: Marian Chace Memorial Fund of the American Dance Therapy Association.

Chodorow, J. (1986). The body as symbol: Dance/movement in analysis. In N. Schwartz-Salant & M. Stein (Eds.), *The body in analysis* (pp. 87–108). Wilmette, IL: Chiron.

Davis, M., Cruz, R., & Berger, M. (1995, August). *Movement and psychodiagnosis: Schizophrenia spectrum and dramatic personality disorders.* Paper presented at the annual conference of the American Psychological Association, New York.

Dosamantes Beaudry, I. (1984). Experiential movement psychotherapy. In P. Lewis (Ed.), *Theoretical approaches in dance/movement therapy* (Vol. 2, pp. 145–163). Dubuque, IA: Kendall/Hunt.

Dosamantes Beaudry, I. (1997). Revisioning dance/movement therapy. *American Journal of Dance Therapy, 19*(1), 16–23.

Espenak, L. (1981). *Dance therapy: Theory and application.* Springfield, IL: Thomas.

Feder, B., & Feder, E. (1998). *The art and science of evaluation in the arts therapies: How do you know what's working?* Springfield, IL: Thomas.

Jordan, J., Kaplan, A., Miller, J., Stiver, I., & Surrey, L. (1991). *Women's growth in connection: Writings from the Stone Center.* New York: Guilford Press.

Kalish-Weiss, B. (1976). *Body Movement Scale for Autistic and Other Atypical Children: An exploratory study using a normal group and an atypical group.*

Doctoral dissertation, Bryn Mawr College, PA. *Dissertation Abstracts International, 36*(10).

Kestenberg, J. (1975). *Children and parents.* New York: Aronson.

Kestenberg Amighi, J., Loman, S., Lewis, P., & Sossin, M. (1999). *The meaning of movement: Developmental and clinical perspectives of the Kestenberg Movement Profile.* New York: Taylor & Francis.

Kornblum, R. (2002). *Disarming the playground: Violence prevention through movement and pro-social skills.* Oklahoma City, OK: Wood & Barnes.

Levy, F. (1992). *Dance/movement therapy: A healing art* (rev. ed.). Reston, VA: American Alliance for Health, Physical Education, Recreation and Dance.

Levy, F. (1995). *Dance and other expressive art therapies: When words are not enough.* New York: Routledge.

Lewis, P. (1986). Psychodynamic ego psychology in developmental dance–movement therapy. In P. Lewis (Ed.), *Theoretical approaches in dance–movement therapy* (Vol. 1, pp. 133–272). Dubuque, IA: Kendall/Hunt.

Lewis, P. (1996). Depth psychotherapy in dance/movement therapy. *American Journal of Dance Therapy, 18*(2), 95–114.

Lewis, P. (2002). *Integrative holistic health, healing, and transformation: A guide for practitioners, consultants, and administrators.* Springfield, IL: Thomas.

Loman, S. (1994). Attuning to the fetus and young child: Approaches from dance/ movement therapy. *Zero to Three: Bulletin of National Center for Clinical Infant Programs, 15*(1), 20–26.

Loman, S. (1998). Employing a developmental model of movement patterns in dance/movement therapy with young children and their families. *American Journal of Dance Therapy, 20*(2), 101–115.

Loman, S., & Foley, L. (1996). Models for understanding the nonverbal process in relationships. *Arts in Psychotherapy, 23*(4), 341–350.

Loman, S., & Merman, H. (1996). The KMP: A tool for dance/movement therapy. *American Journal of Dance Therapy, 18*(1), 29–52.

Loman, S., & Merman, H. (1999). The KMP as a tool for dance/movement therapy. In J. Kestenberg Amighi, S. Loman, P. Lewis, & K. M. Sossin (Eds.), *The meaning of movement: Developmental and clinical perspectives of the Kestenberg Movement Profile* (pp. 211–234). New York: Taylor & Francis.

Mahler, M., Pine, F., & Bergman, A. (1975). *The psychological birth of the human infant: Symbiosis and individuation.* New York: Basic Books.

Musicant, S. (2001). Authentic movement: Clinical considerations. *American Journal of Dance Therapy, 23*(1), 17–28.

Naess, J. (1982). A developmental approach to the interactive process in dance/ movement therapy. *American Journal of Dance Therapy, 5*, 43–55.

Sandel, S. (1993a). The process of empathic reflection in dance therapy. In S. Sandel, S. Chaiklin, & A. Lohn (Eds.), *Foundations of dance/movement therapy: The life and work of Marian Chace* (pp. 98–111). Columbia, MD: Marian Chace Memorial Fund of the American Dance Therapy Association.

Sandel, S. (1993b). Imagery in dance therapy groups: A developmental approach. In S. Sandel, S. Chaiklin, & A. Lohn (Eds.), *Foundations of dance/movement therapy: The life and work of Marian Chace* (pp. 112–119). Columbia, MD: Marian Chace Memorial Fund of the American Dance Therapy Association.

Siegel, E. (1984). *Dance–movement therapy: Mirror of our selves.* New York: Human Sciences Press.

Stanton-Jones, K. (1992). *An introduction to dance movement in psychiatry.* London: Tavistock/Routledge.

Whitehouse, M. (1986). C. G. Jung and dance therapy: Two major principles. In P. Lewis (Ed.), *Theoretical approaches in dance-movement therapy* (Vol. 1, pp. 61–85). Dubuque, IA: Kendall/Hunt.

Winnicott, D. W. (1965). *The maturational processes and the facilitating environment.* New York: International Universities Press.

✂ 5

Drama Therapy
and Psychodrama

ROBERT J. LANDY

From a developmental point of view, drama begins as an infant becomes aware of his or her body as a separate entity that can be recognized and named. In many ways, the genesis of drama mimics the genesis of consciousness in that through both developing human beings are able to stand outside themselves and view themselves as a separate entity. In observing myself, I become two entities: one who thinks, senses, and names, and another who is thought about, taken in through the senses, and named. In psychological terms, these entities are called "I" and "me" (James, 1950; Mead, 1934). In dramatic terms, these two entities are called "actor" and "role," or "actor" and "observer."

The human ability to dramatize is inborn and unlearned. All human beings engage with their inner lives through thought and with their social lives through action, both of which are dramatic to the extent that there is a separation between the I and the me, the part that thinks or acts and the part that is thought about or acted upon. The most obvious form of drama is the moment when the child takes on a role and pretends to be the other. A young girl, for example, takes on the role of mother at bedtime and says to her favorite teddy bear: "If you don't brush your teeth before going to bed, you'll get cavities."

The natural drama of human existence is often applied to other arenas. Dramatic activity can become theatre, the performance by actors of a text to an audience for aesthetic purposes. It can become educational drama, the application of dramatic approaches to teaching to foster the learning of students. It can become ritual and prayer, as repeated and rehearsed actions provide spiritual and social functions for a particular community of celebrants. Drama is also created in the service of healing. Although shamanic healers have used drama, dance, and chant for many thousands of years in many diverse cultures, this chapter will address relatively recent applications of drama to healing: psychodrama and drama therapy.

HISTORICAL BACKGROUND

Although both applications of drama were developed for therapeutic purposes, each has a unique history. Psychodrama was founded by Jacob Levy Moreno (1889–1974), a Viennese psychiatrist who developed his radical approaches to dramatic healing in the early part of the 20th century. Moreno challenged Freud's notion that effective psychological change occurs primarily through a "talking cure," the verbal exchange between analyst and analysand. For Moreno, change occurred most clearly through dramatic enactment. In his system of psychodrama, the analysand became the protagonist who would replay disturbing experiences in his or her life in front of an audience of peers. The audience served to help the protagonist effectively dramatize a troubling scene and release repressed feelings stimulated in the dramatization. Following the psychodramatic enactment, the group audience would support the protagonist and share their own feelings triggered by the drama.

After Moreno emigrated from Austria to the United States in the 1920s, he founded a center for psychodrama in Beacon, New York, where he developed many of his ideas not only in psychodrama, but also in its social applications: sociodrama, sociometry and group psychotherapy. Moreno was a tireless and prolific innovator who extended his ideas to the fields of media and communications, and to sociological and spiritual concerns.

Moreno and his wife, Zerka, continued to be the primary theorists and practitioners of psychodrama and sociodrama throughout the 20th century. Zerka Moreno actively extends their work into the 21st century. Generations of practitioners have discovered their own applications of psychodrama to play (Blatner, 1996), to religion (Pitzele, 1998), to psychological trauma (Dayton, 1997), to criminal justice (Yablonski, 1992), and to social issues (Sternberg & Garcia, 1994). Related forms of psychodrama have developed, most notably Playback Theatre, a community-based form of story dramatization founded by Jonathan Fox and Jo Salas (Salas, 1993). Further, culturally specific forms of psychodrama have developed in different countries (e.g., Rojas-Bermudez, 1995; Kellermann, 1992). And yet in all these examples the form developed by Moreno remains intact, offering a clear structure to all.

Psychodrama can be defined as a form of action psychotherapy where protagonists play themselves in problematic situations in their lives in front of an audience of peers who assist in the drama and feed back their own personal experiences stimulated by the enactment. *Drama therapy* is also a form of action psychotherapy where individuals play roles, often with others in a group, for therapeutic purposes. However, there are some significant differences between the two forms of dramatic healing:

1. Drama therapy was pioneered by several individuals and has spawned several different approaches.
2. In drama therapy protagonists often work in a fictional frame, a playspace, taking on the roles of people or objects different from themselves, more in keeping with the structure of theatre.
3. Drama therapists tend to work with imaginary stories, sometimes working directly with dramatic texts, again establishing a direct connection to theatre.
4. Drama therapists tend to practice in a more eclectic way, one less tied to a single method.
5. Drama therapists incorporate psychodramatic concepts and methods as part of their treatment strategy.

Two independent strands of drama therapy developed in England and the United States. In England, Peter Slade coined the term *dramatherapy* (one word) in the early 1950s. Slade's therapeutic understanding of drama sprang from his work in educational drama with children (Slade, 1952, 1995). Sue Jennings (1974, 1987, 1990, 1997) was instrumental in defining the parameters of the field and extending its scope within many client populations and training programs throughout the world. In the 1960s, Marion Lindkvist founded Sesame, an important training organization in London, where she introduced her ideas on movement and drama for healing purposes.

Following Slade, Jennings, and Lindkvist, a number of practitioners and theorists have made significant contributions to the development of drama therapy in England and indeed throughout the world: Aldia Gersie (1991, 1992, 1997), Phil Jones (1996), and Roger Grainger (1990, 1995), among many others.

In the United States, several innovators were responsible for initially developing and organizing the profession of drama therapy. Among them were Eleanor Irwin, a child psychoanalyst who began her career as a speech therapist and drama specialist; Gertrud Schattner, an educator and drama therapist; and David Read Johnson, a clinical psychologist and drama therapist.

Through publication, research, and the founding of academic programs and private training institutes, the three most influential pioneers have been Renée Emunah, David Read Johnson, and Robert Landy. Emunah founded the Drama Therapy Program at Antioch College (now California Institute for Integral Studies) and wrote the influential text *Acting for Real* (1994), based upon an eclectic approach to drama therapy, one that incorporates psychodrama. Johnson established an innovative approach to therapeutic enactment, Developmental Transformations, and has developed a training institute, the Institutes for the Arts in Psychotherapy, to support the growth of all the creative arts therapies. I founded the Drama Therapy Program at New York University and developed an approach to dramatic healing based upon the ways and means of taking on and playing out dramatic roles. My approach, as well as the approaches of Emunah and Johnson, are discussed below.

Many other Americans have defined drama therapy in their own fashion. A good cross section of these voices can be found in an excellent anthology edited by Lewis and Johnson (2000). Although the growth of the field is most clearly visible in England and the United States, others continue to innovate in Canada, Israel, the Netherlands, Germany, Italy, and Greece.

MAJOR APPROACHES

This section discusses the classic Morenian approach to psychodrama as well as three major approaches to drama therapy. Each approach is considered from both a theoretical and a practical point of view, when appropriate.

Psychodrama

Moreno, strongly influenced by the metaphor of the world as stage and people as players, worked from the assumption that when people take on a role they reveal aspects of themselves. In fact, in an early publication (Moreno, 1946), he defined *role* as "the actual and tangible forms which the self takes." Although he never fully developed his role theory, he held fast to the idea that individuals in role not only reveal aspects of themselves, but do so in a way that allows them to express and release pent-up emotion and feel more resolved having done so. For Moreno, there are four types of roles:

1. *Psychosomatic or physiological roles,* pertaining to the body. These roles include eater, sleeper, eliminator, and mover.
2. *Psychodramatic or fantasy roles,* pertaining to the imagination. These roles include gods, devils, and animals. They can also include roles that one wishes for, such as those concerning success and power.
3. *Social roles,* based in actual relationships with others. They include family, gender and work-based roles in relationship to others.
4. *Cultural roles,* developing in response to the demands of a particular environment. They point to ways that people will enact their particular gender, family, and work roles.

Moreno (1946) believed that one took on a role in order "to enter the unconscious from the social world and bring shape and order to it." Over many years, Moreno worked with various people in difficult emotional or social circumstances, including prostitutes, homeless children, and schizophrenic adults, and helped them create an inner sense of order through effectively reenacting their social circumstances in his psychodrama theatres.

The goal of psychodrama is to enable people to play their roles in a more spontaneous fashion. Moreno (1946) once described this ability to be spontaneous in theatrical terms, viewing the actor as adding freshness to the literal text of the playwright.

In the service of spontaneity, Moreno developed a clearly delineated approach. Psychodrama is a group modality and the small or larger group (ranging from approximately four to 20 individuals) begins with a warm-up whose purpose is to prepare the group to work creatively and to trigger a specific issue within one or more members of the group. As an example, an empty chair is placed in the center of the room and a name, such as Depression, is given to the chair by the director or group member. All group members are then asked to speak directly to the chair.

Once an individual is warmed up, she is chosen as the protagonist, or central figure in the psychodrama. A woman named Rita, for example, might speak to the Depression chair in a deeply felt way. The experience might remind her of a talk she once had with her mother. When this happens, Rita is warmed up and can be chosen by the director, the group, or by herself as the protagonist.

The next part of the session is called the "action phase" which involves a preparation preceding the actual dramatization. During the preparation, the director works to clarify the scene—for example, an important discussion between mother and daughter—to establish a therapeutic bond with the protagonist, to set some limits for the scene, and to cast others in the group in auxiliary roles. The protagonist will generally choose the group members who will play auxiliary roles in her drama. In the example above, Rita may choose an older woman to play her mother.

Then the director will help the protagonist set the scene for the encounter between mother and daughter on the subject of depression and begin the scene. At the most basic level, the protagonist as daughter and the auxiliary as mother will engage with each other directly. But since the purpose of the psychodrama is to foster spontaneity and promote catharsis or emotional release, the director will employ various techniques to arrive at those goals. Techniques include *doubling*, where a member of the group is chosen by the protagonist as an alter ego to speak out her inner thoughts; *soliloquy*, where the protagonist is asked to speak out her inner thoughts alone, deepening her affect; and *role reversal*, where the protagonist and auxiliary literally change roles and continue the drama. There are many other techniques designed to help the protagonist go deeper and arrive at the heart of the issue being portrayed.

Once the drama has reached a heightened moment, often through emotional catharsis, the final phase of the process occurs, that of sharing. During this phase, the group members engage with the protagonist, helping her to process her dramatized experience. Further, individuals share their own experiences around the common theme of, for example, depression or mother and daughter communication. In their communal sharing, the full group reflects upon the theme and acknowledges its significance in their lives.

Role Theory and Role Method in Drama Therapy

As in psychodrama, role theory in drama therapy begins with the premise that human beings take on and play out roles as a natural means of expression. Like Moreno, I (Landy, 2000) attempt to specify the concept of role. In lieu of a definition, I offer the following understanding:

> Human experience, according to role theory, can be conceptualized in terms of discrete patterns of behavior that suggest a particular way of thinking, feeling or acting. Role is one name for these patterns. Each role, although related to other roles, is unique in terms of its qualities, function and style. Role is not necessarily a fixed entity, but one that is capable of change according to the changing life circumstances of the individual role-player. However, like Jung's notion of archetype, each role is recognizable by virtue of its unique characteristics. For example, when one plays the role of mother, certain discernable qualities will be expressed, including a sense of nurturing and care-taking of another. Although the archetypal nature of the role will remain constant over time, certain specific qualities may change as, for example, one in the mother role expresses the desire to be mothered herself or to abrogate her responsibilities toward her child. Even in the extreme, as a mother engages in fantasies of infanticide, Medea-like, she still maintains the essential qualities of mother. Each role can therefore be identified by its archetypal qualities and its degree of deviation from those qualities, as long as the deviance is understood in relation to the norm. (p. 52)

I (Landy, 1993) point to theatre as the source of role and develop a taxonomy of roles based upon a study of Western dramatic literature from the early Greek drama to contemporary forms. I identify 84 role types and related subtypes, repeated figures found within the history of Western drama, and offer evidence that these theatrical types recapitulate behaviors in role of human beings in both drama therapy and everyday life.

Further, I make the case that the aim of drama therapy treatment is to help people find a balance between their contradictory roles, such as that of the victim and the survivor, and to learn to live with their role ambivalences. The full configuration of roles within any human being, equivalent to the personality structure, is referred to as the "role system" (see Landy, 1993).

Leading from role theory, I specify a practical model through which to work with the roles in the taxonomy. The three-part model is comprised of role, counterrole, and guide. I (Landy, 2000) define each as follows:

> When a client begins drama therapy, the drama therapist working from the point of view of role theory often assumes that at least one role the client needs to play in life is either unavailable, poorly developed or inappropriately aligned with other roles or other people in their roles. The initial task of therapy, then, is to help the client access that role and identify it.
>
> In theatrical terms, the role is the protagonist in the client's drama, even though this figure might not yet be aware of the struggles it will undergo in its search for awareness and connection. The counterrole (CR) is the figure that lurks on the other side of the role, the antagonist. It is not the opposite of the role as evil is to good, but rather other sides of the role that may be denied or avoided or ignored in the ongoing attempt to discover effective ways to play a single role. CR is not necessarily a dark or negative figure. If one plays the social role of mother, the CR might be brother or daughter or father. Or it might be something more particular to a client's issues, like helper. For such a client, mother might represent a punitive or abusive figure.
>
> The CR has no independent existence outside of the role. Role appears to have an independent existence and many clients hope to find a way to enact a given role with a degree of competence. Yet even role seeks connection to its counterparts. To be a truly moral person demands an ability to acknowledge and make peace with the immoral or amoral qualities that lurk on the other side.
>
> Role and CR often shift, so that role reversals occur with some regularity. In struggling with moral issues, a client can choose to work with the role of saint or sinner and allow for a shift as one role moves from foreground to background.
>
> The guide . . . is the final part of the role trinity. The guide is a transitional figure that stands between role and CR and is used by either one as a bridge to the other. One primary function of the guide is integration. Another is to help clients find their own way. As such, the guide is a helmsman, pilot and pathfinder, a helper who leads individuals along the paths they need to follow. In its most basic form, the guide is the therapist. One comes to therapy because there is no effective guide figure available in one's social or intrapsychic world. (p. 53)

Looking at a new way to work with Rita, the drama therapist would help her locate the figures of role and counterrole and attempt to discover a third figure that can stand in as guide. The guide could be a family figure, such as mother or daughter, child or father, or it could be a more abstract figure, such as Depression or Expression. The drama therapist working from this perspective would follow the steps of the role method specified as follows by Landy (2000):

1. Invoking the role.
2. Naming the role.
3. Playing out/working through the role.
4. Exploring relationships of role to counterrole and guide.
5. Reflecting upon the role play: discovering role qualities, functions and styles inherent in the role.
6. Relating the fictional role to everyday life.
7. Integrating roles to create a functional role system.
8. Social modeling: discovering ways that clients' behavior in role affects others in their social environments.

The drama therapist would begin a group with a warm-up, similar to those used in psychodrama. The purpose of the warm-up is to help each individual invoke or locate a role. Once the role is present, the drama therapist asks clients to name the roles and begin to work with them. Through the work, the drama therapist helps them explore counterroles and guide roles. As in psychodrama, the drama therapist might look for a single protagonist who would work with the group to explore her roles. At times, however, the drama therapist will work with the full group simultaneously, looking for ways to find forms through which to explore common group concerns.

Rita's group might be asked to move about the room and let a role figure emerge from their body movements. When asked to name the role, Rita might say: "The daughter." In working with Rita, the drama therapist would ask: "Show us what role is on the other side of the daughter." A mother figure might emerge and then perhaps a guide figure, such as Depression or Expression, all of whom would be played out in the group. Following the enactment, the therapist would lead the group into a discussion with Rita reflecting upon the meaning of roles enacted and their connection to the everyday life of Rita. Similar to a psychodramatic sharing, group members would support Rita and tell their own personal stories of mothers and daughters, of depression and expression.

Through the enactments and the reflections in drama therapy, the therapist aims toward helping individuals and groups discover a balance and integration among their roles. For many seeking therapy, an effective guide role is absent or at least illusive. The work then serves to help people construct and internalize guide figures who can enable them to hold their roles and counterroles together. For Rita, it may be that in confronting her mother's depression, she is able to accept a painful legacy left to her by her mother and move toward a more effective way of mothering herself and her own daughter. It may be that in the dramatic enactments Rita is able to reconceive Depression, a negative guide, through the more positive counterfigure of Expression.

The final phase of the role method is social modeling. When one person in a group is changed, she affects all others. As Rita becomes a stronger mother, daughter, and expressive being, she will present a positive model for others in her therapy group, in her family, and in other groups.

The Integrative Five-Phase Model of Drama Therapy

Renée Emunah (1994) also offers a practical model of treatment based in specific stages, or phases. The model incorporates an understanding and application of role theory as well as psychodrama. It also includes reference to dramatic play, theatre, and dramatic ritual. As Emunah presents a model based more solidly in practice rather than in theory, my discussion will be centered on its practical aspects. However, Emunah (2000) does mention that her model is based in humanistic psychology, most especially the work of Rogers and Maslow, with some attention to concepts from existential, psychodynamic, and cognitive-behavioral approaches.

Phase One is that of *dramatic play*. For Emunah, dramatic play is the basic building block that supports all subsequent phases. As in psychodrama, dramatic play fosters spontaneity and leads to the development of positive social interactions among the participants. Dramatic play is improvisational—that is, made up by participants in the moment—and includes such activities as dramatic exercises, creative dramatics, and theatre games. Through the dramatic play, the participants warm up to their creativity and playfulness and develop a level of group trust. Dramatic play activities can be structured or unstructured, depending upon the needs of an individual or group.

In Phase Two, that of *scenework*, participants begin to develop "sustained dramatic scenes, composed of developed roles and characters" (Emunah, 2000, p. 74). Generally speaking, participants work through fictional roles, which differentiates this approach from psychodrama. Their scenes tend to be improvised, although some drama therapists work with scripted stories or plays, if they are germane to a specific group issue. During Phase Two, clients begin to comment upon the themes and roles they have played, connecting the fiction of the drama to their everyday lives, as in Step 6 of Landy's role model. At the end of Phase Two, the audience or clients observing the scenework offer their own reflections, a process similar to the sharing that occurs during the closure period of a psychodrama session. For Emunah, it is important for the drama therapist to help clients maintain the fictional frame in Phases One and Two in order to experience a sense of safety in revealing aspects of themselves.

Role play is the focus of Phase Three. According to Emunah (2000, p. 75), "Central to Phase Three is the notion of drama as rehearsal for life." Through role play, clients shift from the fictional mode to the everyday mode and examine specific problems or issues in their lives such as losing a job, expressing disappointment to a friend, or completing an unfinished conversation with a parent. In role play, clients prepare for job interviews, important conversations, and presentations. Emunah notes that this phase is informed by role theory and that one central aim for clients is to develop a greater awareness of their repertory of roles and of the quality of their role playing in everyday life.

In Phase Three, clients engage in psychodramatic role reversal, playing not only themselves, but also significant others. For example, Rita might be asked to take on the role of her mother and play out a scene with another group member in the role of Rita. The emphasis in Phase Three is on playing with alternative forms of behavior and discovering new ways of responding to old, often embedded, situations. For example, as Rita discovers more about her mother's point of view, she has the potential to alter her behavior in relationship to her mother and to speak to her in a more personally meaningful way.

Phase Four is that of *culminating enactment*. This phase is marked by a shift from behavior to a deeper revelation of core issues. This shift moves the individual into a more introspective mode and proceeds more directly through psychodramatic processes. According to Emunah (2000), "There is an increased focus on the individual within the group, as the inner lives of protagonists are dramatically explored and their stories revealed" (p. 77). Emunah sees culminating enactments as more theatrically based than psychodrama in that the clients have developed competency as actors, sometimes creating well-rehearsed dramas she calls "self-revelatory performances." Further, she urges therapists to move toward culminating enactments *only* within an ongoing, supportive group process, as these scenes are climatic points in the group process and require a great deal of support. In creating a performance about her struggle to accept the legacy of depression passed on to her by her mother, Rita would hope to discover a sense not only of acknowledgment by the group, but also of acceptance and exoneration.

The final phase is that of *dramatic ritual*. This Phase Five concerns closure, the transition from the dramatic reality to that of everyday reality, from the safety and support of the therapeutic group to the more unpredictable social interactions of the outside world. Emunah calls this phase "ritual" because it marks a transition in the lives of the group members. It also marks a sense of shared community, a distinguishing factor of all ritual activity. Following the intensity of an extended drama therapy process, a sense of intimacy has been established. This connectedness can be well symbolized through dramatic ritual. Phase Five activities can include group expressions in movement, sound, and story, through image and metaphor, all in the service of validating the significance of the group process and each individual contribution to it.

Developmental Transformations

David Read Johnson (2000) defines developmental transformations as "embodied encounter in the playspace." Johnson's approach is based upon an application of the dynamics of free play to the treatment of individuals and groups through drama therapy. Developmental transformations is a purely improvisational approach where client and therapist interact dramatically within a space that is defined by both as a place to play, an environment that is dramatic in its separation from everyday reality.

Within the playspace, the client begins to play and the therapist joins in. As players, both allow their roles and the themes of the play to emerge and to change as the natural flow of the action develops. According to Johnson (2000), "The process of play is used to loosen or remove . . . psychic structures that inhibit the client(s) from accessing primary experiences of Being . . ., and the client's progress in treatment is believed to follow natural, developmental processes that in themselves will lead to greater emotional health" (p. 87).

Although based on a number of theoretical approaches in developmental psychology and object relations, Johnson (Johnson, Forrester, Dintino, James, & Schnee, 1996) views his major source as Jerzy Grotowski, who developed the elegant premise that the actor's presence through body and voice is the most essential element in the art form of theatre.

Like psychodrama, developmental transformations concerns the enhancement of spontaneity. Johnson sees the goal as "flow," a concept close in definition to Moreno's understanding of "spontaneity." As in role theory, developmental transformations also aims toward enabling clients to become aware of and to further develop the quality and quantity of their everyday roles. And like Emunah, Johnson believes that the healing progresses through a number of developmental processes, if not phases. Johnson defines several developmental phases in his work: *surface play*, involving the depiction of social stereotypes; *persona play*, involving the depiction of stories from clients' inner and social lives; *intimate play*, involving the depiction of feelings about the therapist; and *deep play*, involving an awareness of the complexity of the human condition as made manifest in the relationship between therapist and client.

Unlike psychodrama, developmental transformations is highly fluid, engaging both client and therapist directly in the creative therapeutic process. At times, there is little distance between the two and the therapist needs to take a time-out, moving into a "witness circle" to observe the play of the client. And like psychodrama, developmental transformations can be highly cathartic as the therapist provokes and encourages the client to express feelings through the body. For Rita, this might be highly energizing, helping her to move from depression to expression through her sound and movement and shifting role plays.

Unlike role theory, developmental transformations is based upon the premise that the healing occurs fully within the enactment. There is no formal reflection following the enactment. When the therapist says "Take a minute," he signals the end of the session. And like role method, developmental transformations attempts first to uncover the ways and means individuals construct and play out their roles, and then to help them deconstruct and reconstruct more effective ways to lead a balanced existence.

Unlike the five phase method, developmental transformations stays with and explores the complex values of dramatic play, without the need to move into a culminating enactment. But like the five phase method, developmental transformations is progressive and epigenetic, building later stages upon earlier ones.

ASSESSMENT AND EVALUATION

Alice Forrester (2000) has effectively reviewed the literature on psychological assessment through role playing and improvisation. Forrester reminds us that dramatic forms of psychological assessment have been in place since World War II. During the 1940s, Henry Murray and his colleagues developed a test for the Office of Strategic Services to measure the readiness of individuals to assume officer rank in the military (see McReynolds & DeVoge, 1977).

Around the same time, Moreno (1946) developed the Spontaneity Test as a means of assessing the ability of clients to engage in spontaneous role play. Because Moreno did not publish very much about the test and its results, we have little evidence about its efficacy.

Throughout the 1970s and 1980s, several cognitive-behavioral approaches to assessment through role play were developed by Kendall (1984), Bandura (1977), and Bandura and Adams (1977). Working within more conventional psychological frameworks, these researchers remained apart from the psychodramatic work of Moreno.

Forrester also refers to a significant drama therapy assessment instrument, the Diagnostic Role-Playing Test (DRPT), developed in the 1970s by David Read Johnson. The test has been used with a number of populations over the years including schizophrenics (see Johnson & Quinlan, 1993), Vietnam War veterans (see James & Johnson, 1997), and normal/neurotic adults. It has also been used as a screening procedure for applicants to a graduate drama therapy program.

In the DRPT subjects are given a series of tasks and are videotaped by the tester, who does not interact with the subjects while they are in action. The DRPT has two parts. In the first test, DRPT 1, a subject is asked to enact five social roles, one at a time: grandparent, bum, politician, teacher, and lover. The subject is presented with 12 props and told to use them in any way she wishes. These props are a wastebasket, a table, a chair, a stick, a cloth, a piece of paper, a cup, a book, a hat, a telephone, a man's overcoat, and a woman's dress. The subject is told: "I am going to ask you to act out five separate roles, one at a time. In each case, show me what these people do . . . " (Johnson, 1988, p. 25).

In the DRPT 2, no props or specific roles are given. The focus is upon the subject's ability to handle interpersonal interaction. The tester gives the following instructions to the subject:

"I am now going to ask you to do three scenes. After each one I will ask you some questions. . . . Enact a scene between three beings in any way that you wish. Who or what these three beings are is up to you. Tell me when you are finished" [See Johnson, 1988, p. 26].

Following each scene the tester asks these questions: "Tell me in as much detail as you can what happened in that scene. . . . Now, describe the three beings, one at a time" (Johnson, 1988, p. 26).

In interpreting both versions of the DRPT, Johnson (1988) adapts aspects of his drama therapy approach to assess the following elements of the subject's role playing:

1. Spontaneity
2. Ability to transcend reality
3. Role repertoire
4. Organization of scenes
5. Patterns in the dramatic content of scenes
6. Attitude toward enactment
7. Style of role playing

Johnson (1988) adds further developmental concepts to aid in interpretation. They include structure of space, task and role, media of representation, complexity of characters and settings, and degree and form of affect.

Eleanor Irwin (1985), a psychoanalytically trained drama therapist, developed another drama therapy approach to assessment through puppetry. Through this approach, called the "Puppet Interview," a child is presented with a basket of puppets and asked to choose one or more. The tester interviews the puppets to learn on one level about the child's perceptions of the puppets, and on a more psychodynamic level the child's perceptions of him- or herself as projected onto the puppets. Then the child is asked to create a puppet show, followed by a reflective discussion with the tester. Irwin applies psychoanalytic criteria in assessing the form and content of the children's puppet shows and reflective comments.

Since 1997, Landy has been developing two dramatic assessment instruments, Tell-A-Story (TAS) and Role Profiles. Both are based in a role theory framework. Role Profiles was developed initially as a means of extending the Taxonomy of Roles (see Landy, 1993) into clinical assessment. Originally TAS was part of Role Profiles. As Landy refined his attempt to assess a client's role system, TAS became an independent test. Through TAS, Landy aims to assess an individual's ability to invoke roles within a story structure, to discover their meanings within the story, and to link the fictional roles to those in the individual's everyday life.

In TAS, the tester provides the following instructions:

"I would like you to tell me a story. The story can be based upon something that happened to you or to somebody else in real life or it can be completely made-up. The story must have at least one character [see Landy, 2001, p. 131]."

If the subject is unable to tell the story verbally, then she is encouraged to tell it nonverbally, either through sound and movement or with projective objects, such as puppets.

Following the story, the tester asks the subject to identify and name the characters and/or significant objects in the story. Then the subject is asked to specify their qualities, function, and style. The tester also inquires about the theme of the story. Finally, the tester asks the subject to explore connections between the fictional characters and her everyday life.

Role Profiles is a more structured test that involves the sorting of 70 index cards, each of which contains the name of a role, into categories. The tester provides the following instructions:

"This experience is intended to explore your personality as if it were made up characters commonly found in plays, movies, and stories. You will be given a stack of cards. On each card is the name of a role, which is a type of character you have probably seen in movies and plays or read about in stories. Please shuffle the cards thoroughly. Place each card in one of four groups that best describes how you feel about yourself right now. Each group is labeled by a large card which says: I Am This, I Am Not This, I Am Not Sure If I Am This, and I Want To Be This. Try to group the cards as quickly as possible. . . . "

The 70 role cards are as follows:

1. Child	9. Beauty	17. Wise person
2. Adolescent	10. Beast	18. Innocent
3. Adult	11. Average person	19. Villain
4. Elder	12. Sick person	20. Victim
5. Asexual	13. Healer	21. Bigot
6. Homosexual	14. Simpleton	22. Avenger
7. Heterosexual	15. Clown	23. Helper
8. Bisexual	16. Critic	24. Miser

25. Coward	41. Son	57. Killer
26. Survivor	42. Sister	58. Suicide
27. Zombie	43. Brother	59. Hero
28. Lost one	44. Orphan	60. Visionary
29. Pessimist	45. Conservative	61. Sinner
30. Worrier	46. Radical	62. Person of faith
31. Optimist	47. Outcast	63. Atheist
32. Angry person	48. Judge	64. Spiritual leader
33. Rebel	49. Witness	65. God
34. Lover	50. Homeless person	66. Saint
35. Egotist	51. Poor person	67. Demon
36. Mother	52. Rich person	68. Magician
37. Father	53. Warrior	69. Artist
38. Wife	54. Bully	70. Dreamer
39. Husband	55. Slave	
40. Daughter	56. Police	

Following the card sort, the subject is asked a series of questions and led into a discussion to aid the tester in assessing the subject's ability to invoke and attribute meaning to roles and to strive toward a balance among the roles.

Role Profiles has been applied to assessments with a number of groups including normal/neurotics (Landy, Luck, Conner, & McMullian, 2003), pedophiles (Tangorra, 1997), and schizophrenics (Landy et al., 2003). Like other drama therapy assessments, Role Profiles needs to be subjected to further clinical trials and tests of reliability, validity, and generalizability.

PSYCHODRAMA AND DRAMA THERAPY IN PRACTICE

Psychodrama has been around for a good part of the 20th century and will presumably flourish into the 21st. Psychodrama has a tradition of treating mentally ill individuals in Moreno's psychodrama institute in Beacon, New York, and in such psychiatric facilities as St. Elizabeths Hospital in Washington, DC. Psychodramatists have done important work with alcoholic and substance abuse patients in such places as the Caron Foundation and Four Winds Hospital, both in several locations in the Northeast. Others have applied their work to those diagnosed with posttraumatic stress disorder, sexual and physical abuse, and many other disorders.

Although Moreno began his early experimentation with children and social misfits, his work has become more readily associated with groups of adults who have difficulty expressing their feelings and are in need of approaches to help them move beyond intellectual and rational ways of making meaning.

Psychodrama is most often practiced as a group modality, dependent upon an audience of peers to assume auxiliary roles in a protagonist's drama and to share their thoughts and feelings toward the end of a session.

Drama therapy, like psychodrama, has been used in the treatment of a variety of clients from normal neurotic to schizophrenic. Drama therapy, however, is also used with younger populations who are developmentally unprepared to enact complex scenes and reflect upon them in a verbal way. In fact, the earliest form of drama therapy, developmentally speaking, is play therapy, where the therapist engages with the child to elicit a language of images expressed indirectly in the play. Drama therapists have successfully treated young people who have experienced physical and sexual abuse.

Drama therapists also often work with the other side of the developmental spectrum, that is, with elderly clients, some of whom suffer from dementia and Alzheimer's disease. Some of the most challenging and effective work in drama therapy has occurred with homeless mentally ill adults (Schnee, 1996), Vietnam War veterans (James & Johnson, 1997), and young people with various forms of emotional disturbances.

Drama therapy, although primarily practiced in groups, is also used as a form of individual treatment. This can be the case when engaging in the interactive play of developmental transformations, the more client-centered storymaking and role playing of the role method, or the eclectic five phase method.

Although drama therapists make use of psychodramatic principles and techniques, the most unique feature of drama therapy is its projective nature. By that I mean that drama therapists often help clients move into fictional roles within the playspace in order to provide a measure of distance from everyday reality. There are various projective techniques available to all drama therapists including puppets and dolls, masks and makeup, costumes and props, storytelling, sandplay, playmaking, and role playing of all kinds. As an example of a drama therapy session that employs a number of these projective approaches, I present the case of

Wade, a 6-year-old boy living in a residential treatment center for children with varying degrees of behavioral and emotional problems.

I only had the opportunity to do one 60-minute session with Wade. We meet in the playroom, which was equipped with puppets and dolls, costumes and props, many varieties of toys and games, and a large sandbox, about 4 feet by 5 feet. Wade had been living with a number of emotional challenges, including the diagnosis of ADHD and the effects of a broken family, highlighted by a feeling of abandonment from his mother. He was referred to the center for acting out inappropriately and aggressively both in school and at home. At the time of our meeting, Wade had been living with his father. His 10-year-old sister was living with his mother. He had been in residence at the treatment center for 1 week and would stay an additional 2 weeks.

Early in our session, Wade tested me in various ways, trying to determine if I would be a safe and reliable partner in play. He would offer me props and invite me to play with him, which I would do eagerly, setting appropriate boundaries when necessary. He would attempt to run out of the playroom from time to time, and I would cajole him back, offering him the psychological space he needed in the room.

In our initial warm-up play, I attempted to help him identity and name dramatic roles. Shortly thereafter, Wade found a woman's dress and gave it to me. At the same time he discovered a container of stage makeup and proceeded to make himself up as a woman. I was mindful of his intense issues around his rejection by his mother. Further, his primary therapist had also told me that Wade was struggling with his sexual identity. When he asked me to put on the dress, I faced a dilemma. On the one hand, I thought it might be a good idea to take on the role of the mother and to encourage him as son to engage with me. On the other hand, I thought this direct level of role play and potential role reversal might be too stimulating, so I chose to redirect the feminine roles and transform them into more playful and neutral ones.

Luckily, the dress was too small for me to wear so I draped it over my shoulders like a cape. As Wade began to apply makeup, I sat down with him and offered to participate. I asked him who he wanted to be. He responded by dabbing a bit of red greasepaint on my cheek. I laughed and he was pleased, adding more of the paint to his own cheeks. Pretty soon we both had colorful faces and I asked him: "Who are we?"

"Clowns," he replied, and we were safe to play in our new roles. We were off and running, performing tricks, telling jokes, and singing funny songs—all in the service of establishing a strong, safe connection.

At one point, Wade took up a Slinky and held it to his mouth, speaking into it as if it were a megaphone. He gave me the other end and I put it to my ear, eager to learn of his pronouncements. He extended it to its full length and let it fly, hitting me in the ear. I let him know that he had gone too far and that in our play we must keep each other safe from physical harm. He accepted the setting of a safe boundary, and we were ready to proceed to the next, more challenging, roles in our play.

Wade moved from clown to warrior, picking up several weapons along the way: a soft bat, a three-pronged plastic trident, a clothes hanger, and the ever-present Slinky. When I asked him to tell me about the weapons, he told me that he had to defend himself from the witch. At this point, Wade began to set up an elaborate scene in the sandbox. He discovered a family of puppets: father, mother, and two children, one a baby. They were constructed of malleable rubber and were hollow in the center. He planted the puppets in the sand, with the female figure as the most prominent. He identified this figure as the witch and made it clear that she was very wicked and very powerful.

As he gathered the weapons and summoned his strength to fight the witch, he recognized the dangers and difficulty of the task. This was not only a witch, but the most powerful figure in the family of puppets. As a potential representation of his rejecting mother, this witch was a formidable foe.

Wade needed an army or at least a guide. And so I offered to help, accompanying him on the search for weapons and keeping a running commentary going: "We need to make sure that we prepare ourselves. We shouldn't approach a powerful figure until we feel strong enough." At some point, Wade impulsively lunged at the box to kill the evil witch. Not feeling that he was sufficiently prepared internally and fearing a facile and violent solution to a complex moral problem, I intervened: "Maybe she's not all bad. What if the witch has just a little good in her heart?" He responded by backing off and circling the sandbox cautiously. I followed right behind him, my clothes hanger and bat at the ready.

Finally prepared, Wade approached the sandbox and swiped at the witch figure with his clothes hanger several times, with some restraint, until he knocked her over. He gestured for me to join in. Following his lead, I hit her with considerable restraint, and then Wade and I proceeded to knock over the entire family: father, sister, baby in order. When we had completed our mission, Wade put down his weapons, and I did the same. He surveyed the damage and then he took up the family of puppets one by one and began to fill them up with sand. I tried to conceal my astonishment as Wade invited me to join in. We were no longer warriors. We were restorers, healers filling up the wounded family.

As we concluded our work and approached the end of the session, I asked Wade how he felt about the witch. He replied: "I don't think she is a witch anymore. She's a lady with a heart."

When the session was over, Wade bolted out of the room, without saying another word. In the evening, he attended a group therapy session with his father. The next day, his father reported that Wade appeared to be much calmer and less anxious. His primary therapist reported the same. His behavior in school modified as he became less aggressive and more prepared to resume academic tasks.

When Wade left the residence he continued in play therapy, a support he needed to find ways to forgive his mother, reconnect with his family, and build a more positive self-concept. His drama therapy session proved significant in that for the first time he felt empowered to confront the negative mother figure/witch that had so hurt him and to transform her into a figure full of feeling and worthy of compassion.

ANALYSIS

Wade took on several roles in our drama therapy work together: woman, clown, warrior, and healer. After much testing of me, he decided that I might become a reliable guide on his search to find and change the source of his discomfort. As guide, I helped him to locate the counterroles that I felt would help him not only reach his goal, but also better integrate conflicting feelings.

The counterrole of the woman became the clown, the more distanced figure that also wears makeup and behaves in absurd and often incomprehensible ways. In working as clowns, we were both better able to approach the fearful object of the mother without actually taking on that role. By transforming mother to clown, I felt that Wade and I would be safer to proceed on our journey. All throughout I kept looking for ways to build safe roles through which to approach a very difficult and unsafe figure.

The counterrole of the clown became the warrior, the one whose function was to directly fight the enemy. Once Wade was in this role, he was prepared to do battle with the witch/mother. As the warrior, Wade made sure that he armed himself, but with safe weapons of Slinky, clothes hanger, and soft bat, the kinds of weapons a clown would use. This was not to be a real battle but a play battle that would lead to a significant psychological victory.

With each shift of role, Wade was trying to find ways to defeat the ultimate counterrole, the witch, a representation of the fearful mother who had abandoned him. In the end, having well prepared himself with the aid of his guide, he was able to find the right combinations of roles to do the job. In an elegant maneuver, Wade re-created his family as four puppets in a sandbox. In control, he knocked down the witch/ mother, the father, the sister, and the baby—a figure he later identified as himself. And then, taking on a counterrole of the warrior, in the figure of the restorer or healer, he reconstructed that which he had destroyed. In filling up the mother with sand, he gave her new substance. In speaking about his action, he noted that she too had transformed from witch to lady and that her hollowness had been replaced by a heart, the source of feeling. As he filled up all of the family figures, he symbolically reconstructed the whole family that had been so empty in their separation from each other.

Although I stayed with Wade throughout, in many ways guiding his playful heroic journey, in the end he became his own guide, having instigated the filling up of the family, and reflected upon the transformation.

In my work with Wade, I proceeded through many of the steps of the role method. We began by invoking a role, that of woman, which transformed to that of clown and finally to those of warrior and healer. Although this work was not in the strict sense developmental transformations, it had some of the qualities of that approach as Wade and I moved in and out of roles.

Through our work, I attempted to help Wade name his roles, some of which he did, such as clown and witch. In his play, Wade was able to identify and work through his conflict with his family and especially with his mother, represented by the figure of the witch. As he moved from role to counterrole he fluidly explored many interrelationships. He made good use of an external guide figure, the therapist, to help him approach the object of his greatest fear.

Wade was quite verbal and capable of reflecting upon his play verbally. However, he was only 6 years old and in my opinion had worked deeply on an important issue in his life. Although it did not seem necessary to talk much about the play, Wade was well able to verbalize an awareness of the transformation of the evil witch to the feeling mother, a significant reflection. As Wade's behavior became more contained at home and at school, he became a social model for his sister and parents, who themselves needed to create a greater sense of order in their lives.

OTHER APPLICATIONS

In crisis, drama therapy is often an effective approach with children, either in individual or group treatment. After the terrorist attacks on the United States on September 11, 2001, many children experienced an immediate sense of crisis. One boy who lost both his parents in the World Trade Center reacted to the trauma by acting out aggressively, in a more overt and hostile way than Wade did when faced with rejection by his mother. The 10-year-old boy, whom I will call Joe, was inconsolable. His therapist, trained in drama therapy, had the idea of providing a sandtray and miniature objects, similar to those used by Wade. Joe immediately gravitated to the sandtray, took up a handful of soldier and firemen figures, and then buried them in the sand. He proceeded with great concentration and focus until he had finished. When the therapist questioned him as to his next move, without hesitation he began to search for the buried figures, uncovering them one by one, brushing their bodies free of sand, and placing them back on the shelves.

Like Wade, Joe seemed more at ease after this exercise. By indirectly enacting the dreaded rituals he had seen on television and heard in fragmented bits of conversations, he gained a certain understanding and mastery. In the role of the victim, he felt lost and confused. In the counterrole of the rescuer, he felt more in control. The therapist again served as a guide figure, leading him to the imaginary playspace upon which he could work out his troubling drama.

When the tragedy first hit Lower Manhattan, I engaged in crisis counseling with a number of adults. Unlike the children, they did not have the need to play out their horrific experiences indirectly. All needed in the most direct way to tell their stories. The stories were highly various as to point of view. Some escaped from the World Trade Center Towers, others were evacuated from nearby buildings, still others watched the full drama from their apartments, homes, and backyards. Some heard of the events in disbelief while in transit to work or at the workplace. Some lost loved ones and acquaintances. Others knew of those lost. Some, not knowing anyone lost directly, mourned the dead and their own sense of helplessness equally.

As I listened to the stories, I noted some common roles and counterroles: villains, victims, and heroes; helpless ones and helpers;

fundamentalists and tolerant ones; hawks and doves. Each storyteller yearned for understanding, some for revenge, most for healing. And in the service of healing, I noted that the most important role in all the stories was that of the storyteller. In crisis and trauma, people need to tell their stories, and after September 11, 2001, New York became a city of storytellers.

On the other side of the storyteller is the one who remains silent, attempting to repress the horrific events. Through the process of drama therapy following this tragedy, people in groups met to rise above the counterrole and to express the range of their often confused emotions. This was not psychodrama and not a specific form of drama therapy. It was, rather, a most elemental form of group expression, a ritual narration for the purpose of creating a supportive community and releasing feelings of fear for themselves and pity for those victimized.

I led several groups throughout the weeks that followed September 11. As I listened to more stories, I noted that on the other side of the storyteller was not only the repressed one, but the witness, the one able to listen and to contain, to acknowledge the significance of the story told by the storyteller. The role of witness was a guiding role throughout all these groups, one that held together the need to tell and the counterneed to repress. As we witnessed each other's stories, we built small communities of survivors with a mission—to listen and to stay as open as possible until all the buried stories were uncovered like the soldiers in the sandbox.

In one group of adults 2 weeks after the attack, several were ready to move from the reality of the stories to imaginary enactment. They created an improvisational drama. One played the role of a teacher and the others her young students. The teacher asked the children to show how they felt about the attacks on the World Trade Center. Several students built two tall buildings with their bodies and several others played airplanes. The planes crashed into the buildings and they all fell down, laughing in a heap on the floor. The teacher congratulated them on their enactment and all were pleased.

When out of role, the adults reflected upon their role play. It was hard to let go in the days following the terrorist attacks, they said. They felt scared and confused. Some felt abandoned by traditional guide figures: political leaders, clergy, God, and even their own rational expectations. Their everyday work and family roles felt difficult to play out effectively. In taking on the role of children, they reexperienced these feelings of loss and through their play were able to let them go.

For some, the child role felt like a guide, a figure that could play with abandon and hold together the seemingly contradictory roles of victim and survivor. In playing out their version of "London Bridge Is Falling Down" as children, the group released its anxiety as generations of others have done before them, finding a meaningful way to calm their fears of succumbing to plagues and bombings and endless forms of man's inhumanity to man.

CONCLUSION

Dramatic experience traverses a wide spectrum from the natural play of children through the formal theatrical presentations of actors. In its application to healing through psychodrama and drama therapy, drama moves toward an inevitable goal. In playing with our contradictions, in giving voice to and letting go of our pain, in searching for effective guide figures, we move closer to balance.

From the classical tragedies we learn that after the demise of both villain and hero, after the destruction of the old order, a new order is established. Chaos is just one pole of the pendulum that swings back to order and balance. The point of healing through drama is that in playing out the chaos of our inner lives and outer realities, a new order emerges. As we find the balance we also find the balancer, the guide principle that holds together the chaos and the order, the role and the counterrole.

REFERENCES

Bandura, A. (1977). Social foundations of thought and action. Englewood Cliffs, NJ: Prentice-Hall.

Bandura, A., & Adams, N. E. (1977). Analysis of self-efficacy theory of behavioral change. Cognitive Theory Research, 1, 287–310.

Blatner, A. (1996). Acting-in: Practical applications of psychodramatic methods (3rd ed.). New York: Springer.

Dayton, T. (1997). Heartwounds: The impact of unresolved trauma and grief on relationships. Deerfield Beach, FL: Health Communications.

Emunah, R. (1994). Acting for real—Drama therapy process, technique, and performance. New York: Brunner/Mazel.

Emunah, R. (2000). The integrative five phase model of drama therapy. In P. Lewis & D. R. Johnson (Eds.), Current approaches in drama therapy (pp. 70–86). Springfield, IL: Thomas.

Forrester, A. (2000). Role-playing and dramatic improvisation as an assessment tool. The Arts in Psychotherapy, 27, 235–243.

Gersie, A. (1991). *Storymaking in bereavement.* London: Kingsley.
Gersie, A. (1992). *Earth tales.* London: Green Press.
Gersie, A. (1997). *Reflections on therapeutic storymaking.* London: Kingsley.
Grainger, R. (1990). *Drama and healing: The roots of dramatherapy.* London: Kingsley.
Grainger, R. (1995). *The glass of heaven—The faith of the dramatherapist.* London: Kingsley.
Irwin, E. (1985). Puppets in therapy: An assessment procedure. *American Journal of Psychotherapy, 39,* 389–400.
James, M., & Johnson, D. R. (1997). Drama therapy in the treatment of combat-related post-traumatic stress disorder. *The Arts in Psychotherapy, 23*(5), 383–395.
James, W. (1950). *The principles of psychology.* New York: Dover Books.
Jennings, S. (1974). *Remedial drama.* London: Pitman.
Jennings, S. (Ed.). (1987). *Dramatherapy: Theory and practice for teachers and clinicians* (Vol. 1). London: Routledge.
Jennings, S. (1990). *Dramatherapy with families, groups and individuals: Waiting in the wings.* London: Kingsley.
Jennings, S. (1997). *Introduction to dramatherapy: Ariadne's ball of thread.* London: Kingsley.
Johnson, D. R. (1988). The diagnostic role-playing test. *The Arts in Psychotherapy, 15,* 23–36.
Johnson, D. R. (2000). Developmental transformations: Toward the body as presence. In P. Lewis & D. R. Johnson (Eds.), *Current approaches in drama therapy* (pp. 87–110). Springfield, IL: Thomas.
Johnson, D. R., Forrester, A., Dintino, C., James, M., & Schnee, G. (1996). Towards a poor drama therapy. *The Arts in Psychotherapy, 23*(4), 293–306.
Johnson, D. R., & Quinlan, D. (1993). Can the mental representations of paranoid schizophrenics be differentiated from those of normals? *Journal of Personality Assessment, 60,* 588–601.
Jones, P. (1996). *Drama as therapy, theatre as living.* London: Routledge.
Kellermann, P. (1992). *Focus on psychodrama: The therapeutic aspects of psychodrama.* London: Kingsley.
Kendall, P. C. (1984). Behavioral assessment and methodology. *American Review of Behavioral Therapy: Theory and Practice, 10,* 47–86.
Landy, R. (1993). *Persona and performance—The meaning of role in drama, therapy, and everyday life.* New York: Guilford Press.
Landy, R. (2000). Role theory and the role method of drama therapy. In P. Lewis & D. R. Johnson (Eds.), *Current approaches in drama therapy* (pp. 50–69). Springfield, IL: Thomas.
Landy, R. (2001). Role profiles—An assessment instrument. In *New essays in drama therapy—Unfinished business* (pp. 144–167). Springfield, IL: Thomas.
Landy, R., Luck, M. B., Conner, E., & McMullian, S. (2003). Role profiles: A drama therapy assessment instrument. *The Arts in Psychotherapy, 30*(3), 151–161.

Lewis, P., & Johnson, D. R. (Eds.). (2000). *Current approaches in drama therapy.* Springfield, IL: Thomas.

McReynolds, P., & DeVoge, S. (1977). Use of improvisational techniques in assessment. In P. McReynolds (Ed.), *Advances in psychological assessment* (Vol. 4, pp. 222–277). San Francisco: Jossey-Bass.

Mead, G. H. (1934). *Mind, self and society.* Chicago: University of Chicago Press.

Moreno, J. L. (1946). *Psychodrama.* New York: Beacon House.

Pitzele, P. (1998). *Scripture windows: Toward a practice of bibliodrama.* Los Angeles: Torah Aura Productions.

Rojas-Bermudez, J. (Ed.). (1995). *Some papers on psychodrama.* Seville, Spain: Association of Psychodrama and Group Psychotherapy.

Salas, J. (1993). *Improvising real life: Personal story in playback theatre.* Dubuque, IA: Kendall/Hunt.

Schnee, G. (1996). Drama therapy in the treatment of the homeless mentally ill. *The Arts in Psychotherapy, 23,* 53–60.

Slade, P. (1954). *Child drama.* London: University Press.

Slade, P. (1995). *Child play.* London: Kingsley.

Sternberg, P., & Garcia, A. (1994). *Sociodrama: Who's in your shoes?* Westport, CT: Praeger.

Tangorra, J. (1997). *Many masks of pedophilia: Drama therapeutic assessment of the pedophile.* Unpublished master's thesis, New York University, New York, NY.

Yablonski, L. (1992). *Psychodrama: Resolving emotional problems through role-playing.* New York: Brunner/Mazel.

6

Poetry Therapy

KENNETH GORELICK

Poetry is the language in which man explores his own
amazement.
—CHRISTOPHER FRY (Fox, 1995, p. 135)

What capacity most distinguishes us as humans: the way we
move, reason, laugh, create, imagine, respond to beauty, manipulate
symbols, devise and use tools, or play? All of them do as a whole. The
arts therapies, each in its unique way, all address these elements of our
humanity. *Poetry therapy* is the intentional application of the written
and the spoken word to growth and healing.

Poetic language is condensed, replete with sensory images, and
charged with meaning. It combines conscious and unconscious dimensions, integrates past–present–future states of being, challenges thought,
stimulates physiological and muscular responses, and resonates with the
paradox and mystery of life. *Poesis,* the Greek root word for the English
poetry, means "calling into existence that which has not existed before."
Poetry therapists use poetic language in all its forms—poem, story, journal, epistle, fable, fairytale, myth, essay, song lyric and chant, even
drama and cinema—in order to help their clients discover the truth of
their own existence, enhance their creative and problem-solving abilities,
communicate and relate better to others, and experience the healing

properties of beauty. Poetry therapists choose for their clients literature written by others designed to provoke and evoke self-understanding. Moreover, they promote clients' self-discovery via their own creative self-expression.

Poetry therapy can be used with clients who are dealing with change and loss, overcoming depression, breaking free of alcohol and drug abuse, mending personal relationships, gaining a better understanding of themselves, and much more.

In general the goals of poetry therapy include:

- Developing an understanding of oneself and others through poetry and other forms of literature.
- Promoting creativity, self-expression, and greater self-esteem.
- Strengthening interpersonal and communication skills.
- Expressing overwhelming emotions and releasing tension.
- Promoting change and increasing coping skills and adaptive functions (National Coalition of Creative Arts Therapies Associations, 2004).

POETRY IN THE CULTURE

People's initial reaction to the word *poetry* may be negatively colored by their contact with English teachers who squeezed the life out of both poetry and students. From the 1920s to the 1950s U.S. poets pursued radical experiments in symbol and abstraction, which cut them and their work off from the average person. But in the last 45 years, thanks to the success of "confessional" poets like Anne Sexton and popular balladeers like Leonard Cohen and Bob Dylan, poetry has returned to its lyrical roots, and once again speaks the language of the heart. Recent poet laureates Robert Haas and Robert Pinsky, the latter with his "Favorite Poems Project," have helped restore poetry as a voice of the people. Gangsta rap, the howl of alienation, makes us squirm. Contemporary bards like Robert Bly, accompanying himself on his lyre, draw enthusiastic audiences. "Poetry slams" generate excitement among youth. Millions have watched the Bill Moyers TV programs on poets and poetry. Poetry books and their readers proliferate. For the poetry therapist and his or her clients, poetry has never been more accessible. But the therapist must sometimes work to undo individuals' negative prior experiences and to open the door to poetry for them.

HISTORY

We may suppose that healing with words began with shamanic incantation.

About 5,000 years ago in what is today Iraq an amazing technological leap was made: a cuneiform picture language engraved on clay tablets was invented. It was the basis for our alphabet.

Some time afterward, Egyptians recorded events of their lives in pharaohs' tombs as a way of ensuring immortality. Magic words written on papyrus were ingested by patients as a cure for disease.

Meanwhile, on the other side of the world, Chinese ideograms were invented. These juxtaposed two or more images, creating an "alphabet" that was visual poetry. The ideogram for "writing" is a turtle poised on the surface of a stream, its engraved shell a permanent record of passing moments. The ideogram for "poetry" (*shih*) is composed of two images: *yen* (language or speaking) and *szu*, (temple). Thus poetry is a temple of words, temple-speaking, or holy.

The *Epic of Gilgamesh*, written three millennia ago, is humankind's first recorded struggle with the pangs of mortality awareness.

Later, that wonderful treasury of tales, the Bible, was written. About 1000 B.C. David healed Saul's melancholy by singing psalms while accompanying himself on the harp.

In fifth-century B.C. Greece, the drama was considered an integral part of communal healing. Theatre portrayed traumas like murder, rape, and incest. It presented the question of fate versus free will in the outcomes of peoples' lives. Aristotle explained the mechanism of "katharsis": the spectator experiences "terror," that is, vicariously takes the role of sufferer, and "pity," that is, vicariously takes the role of healer (Gorelick, 1987).

The record of words as healing agents is continuous. Freud said, "Not I, but the poets, discovered the unconscious." By the late 1940s Caroline Shrodes was applying a psychoanalytic framework to understand how literature impacts the reader's psyche (Shrodes, 1960).

The modern field of poetry therapy was established by psychiatrist Jack Leedy, who started a poetry therapy clinic at Cumberland Hospital in Brooklyn, New York, and issued a call for contributors to a book. His work as an editor (Leedy, 1969, 1973) brought together a critical mass of practitioners from the fields of therapy, education, and literature and launched the first poetry therapy organization, the Association for Poetry Therapy (APT).

Psychologist Arthur Lerner (1994) introduced poetry therapy to two hospitals in the Los Angeles area, established the Poetry Therapy Institute, and inspired many to enter the field.

At St. Elizabeths Hospital in Washington, DC, Arleen Hynes introduced poetry therapy to staff and patients and created an influential training program. She codified training standards for clinical and for developmental poetry therapists and founded the organization that today credentials poetry therapists, the National Federation for Biblio/Poetry Therapy. She also coauthored an unexcelled training manual (Hynes & Hynes-Berry, 1986).

In 1981 Sherry Reiter and others transformed APT into today's membership organization, the National Association for Poetry Therapy (NAPT; website: *www.poetrytherapy.org*). Its annual meetings have included as keynoters nationally prominent poets sympathetic to poetry therapy, including Jimmy Santiago Baca, Rafael Campo, Lucille Clifton, Edward Hirsch, Linda Pastan, Marge Piercy, Naomi Shihab Nye, and Judith Viorst. NAPT sponsors the quarterly *Journal of Poetry Therapy*, which founder Nicholas Mazza has edited since 1986.

In 1993 Peggy Heller founded a nonprofit fundraising arm, the NAPT Foundation, which raises funds for such activities as regional educational meetings, training scholarships, and poetry therapy community projects. It has funded publication of the poetry of Columbine High School survivors and has distributed free of charge *Giving Sorrow Words*, a volume of consolation poems following the 9/11 tragedy. (For more history, see Reiter, 2004, and Morrison, 1982.)

DEVELOPMENTAL MODEL

Poetry therapists attempt to contextualize the client and his or her problem: Where in the life cycle is the client? How did he or she get here? What is the next step? For poetry therapists, "development" means "*language* development."

Young human beings prior to the development of speech are like other animals in communicating needs through their gestures and nonword sounds. Thus they communicate such needs and emotions as hunger, fear, danger, frustration, aggression, excitement, territoriality, recognition of friends and strangers, contentment, the desire to be alone, and the desire for contact. Poetry therapists look and listen for these deep patterns of rhythm and sound lying beneath semantics and syntax to better understand client actions and meanings. The therapist perceives discrepancies between what the client says and what the client feels. For example, clients who are too verbal, too intellectualized, too isolated from feelings and sensations can return to their body via rhythm.

Words are people connectors. Relationship is fundamental in therapy as in life. Language is acquired through the mother–child bond, giving us our "mother tongue." Mothers use a special dialect, what we might call "parentese." They enunciate vowels more slowly, speak at a higher pitch, and use an exaggerated cadence as they communicate with their infants (Kuhl, 2002). As poetry therapists attune to the nuances of clients' language, they invoke the intimacy of the mother–child bond, and they attempt to succor the isolated, the lonely, or the depressed client.

From the beginning of a mother–child relationship, Mom is communicating existential truths about hurt and healing. As she croons in a soothing voice "Rock-a-bye baby in the tree top . . . and when the bough breaks the cradle will fall," she indicates that danger exists, but also that there is safety. As Mom reads " . . . and all the king's horses / and all the king's men / couldn't put Humpty Dumpty together again," baby learns another existential truth: eggs and people break, and sometimes all we can do is bear witness. Poetry therapists help their clients find the words to describe their loss, but they also help them to find words that bring hope.

The infant soon learns the power of words to order the world, perceiving the power of the parents as he begins to call them "Mamma" and "Dada," and to issue commands: "Dimmi." Reality and words have a reciprocal relationship. Reality makes us invent words to characterize events and experience, and words cue us about our culture's reality. Poetry therapists assist clients to rename and reframe their reality, thereby altering it; to perceive their wants and needs, reaching out to attain them.

Words are not mere abstractions: they carry bodily weight. According to Christensen (1986), the rhythms within a poem "constitute a graph of the respiration and metabolic consequences that an experience forces upon the human organism" (p. 97). In rhythm "we hear those fuzzy, water-logged syllables of our mother's speech . . . the murmurs of the universe, our amniotic sea's own voice, pumped through . . . the thick muscular walls surrounding us, the voice of the mother, primordial, distant as thunder, profound, earth-shattering, and sweeter than any other sense in our memory. Vowels [begin to draw the speaker/reader] into the great subhuman depths of nature where the energy of one is the energy of all. . . . In the vowels and their endless, inexhaustible permutations through consonantal context, the human descends into the animal universe once again" (p. 97). Poetry therapists know that words promote actions in our body. Words can be powerful "placebos," with the capability for both therapeutic and toxic effects. Such effects can be very powerful when therapists work with persons recovering from acute somatic illnesses or in trying to slow the progress of chronic ailments.

Bedtime and other stories are part of the rituals of childhood. In the childhood of humanity the tribal storyteller retold creation myths and ancestor tales to build community cohesion and continuity. Still later folk and fairy tales were wisdom carriers. The coarser ones preached "do's and don'ts." The elegant ones inspired the listener's own creativity in meeting life's challenges (Bettelheim, 1977). Today poetry therapists help individuals to "story" their lives, help couples and families to find their story, and help members of organizations to build their work communities.

Poetry therapists believe in the importance of the "now" moment as the axis of possible change. And we believe too in moments unfurling as a spiral of development determined by biological, psychological, and cultural forces. While development is continuous, there are critical periods of flowering for successive life tasks from birth to death (Erikson, 1963). Arts capacities follow this unfolding (Johnson, 1999).

Spiral development means we reencounter old issues time and again, at a familiar, yet different, point. Past, present, and future align in harmonic resonance in the teachable moment of therapeutic encounter. This view leads to a frame that helps guide each session. The participant contacts a poem "out there," takes it in, goes deeper, where it resonates the depths, activates resistances and harmonies, and leads to a resolution of the moment, which is put back "out there," where it is taken up and responded to by others, creating a new "out there," and thereby changing the cosmos ever so slightly (Hynes & Hynes-Berry, 1986; Heller, 1995). Past, present, and future align in harmonic resonance that creates openings for the new.

THERAPEUTIC ACTION: POETRY AS METAPHOR

Poetry contains and unleashes the power of metaphor. It juxtaposes one thing with another, exchanges meanings, and opens up new possibilities and understandings. A *metaphor* is itself and something else at the same time. It enlarges, it connects, it shatters old frameworks (Gorelick, 1989). Metaphor unlocks the meanings inherent in particular objects and ordinary events (Cox & Theilgaard, 1986).

Good metaphors are not abstractions but are quite specific and concrete. They can be touched, felt, tasted. For example, a bottle of maraschino cherries that stood unopened in the fridge throughout childhood contains the essence of that childhood. In contrast to the other items, these cherries were "on fire / lit-from-within red / heart red, sexual red, wet neon red." We feel the pain of unquenched desires—his and our own. And we treat that pain with understanding: "if I never ate one / it was because it might be missed / or because I knew it would not be replaced. . . . " And now words are a way to experience that kick of desire: "because you do not eat / that which rips your heart with joy" (Lux, 1997, "Refrigerator, 1957").

The enduring image can substitute for what has been lost. Contemporary writer Susan Woolridge (1996) describes the therapy of writing about her dying father: "How can my father be captured and held, how can I stave off the upcoming loss but in the possibility of a poem. . . . In a poem I can have him whole. . . . I need to make this poem to my father spiral up, spiral down, catch him and compel me, without him, to love life" (p. 195).

LOVE AND LOSS

Asked what poetry is "about," most people who have studied some poetry would likely say it's "about love and death." In reality, in looking at many, many poems, we find that just about every experience under the sun has been portrayed in poetry. Poems are indeed an enumeration of love and loss, but they are much more: "birds, bees, babies, butterflies, bugs, bambinos, babayagas, and bipeds, beating their way up bewildering bastions" (Sandburg, 1950, "Tentative (First Model) Definitions of Poetry," p. 319). But the undertext really is an attempt to maintain vitality in the face of our existential limitations of finiteness, aloneness, vulnerability, and mortality. Loss shadows every change. Nearly every poem—except some few that bespeak the philosophy of nihilism—affirms life in the face of death. "everything / I have ever learned / in my lifetime / leads back to this: the fires / and the black river of loss / whose other side / is salvation. . . . / To live in this world / you must be able / to do three things: / to love what is mortal; / to hold it / against your bones knowing / your own life depends on it; / and, when the time comes to let it go, / to let it go" (Oliver, 1983, "In Blackwater Woods," p. 82).

THEORETICAL ORIENTATIONS

As a "tool, not a school," poetry therapy integrates the major theoretical orientations summarized below. The schools themselves have recently been converging (Goldfried & Newman, 1986).

Psychoanalytic School

This philosophy proposes that truth is the sufferer's saving grace. Powerful emotions and ancient fears churn continuously within us. Poetry therapy, from this theory, is based on the belief that individuals can grasp and fix what is painful by giving it form. This school of thought uses the dynamic unconscious and techniques that utilize psychodynamic concepts such as transference/countertransference, conflict, and defense and resistance (Alexander & French, 1974).

Interpersonal School

This orientation emphasizes how we co-create one another in relationship. Poetry therapy taking an interpersonal approach uses techniques to help individuals increase their self-understanding in relation to others and uses poetry as a projective screen to see what old scripts we are replaying (Yalom, 1970).

Behavioral/Cognitive School

This approach looks to the power of the rational mind to influence feelings and behaviors. It provides an array of techniques to identify maladaptive patterns and teach new approaches (Taylor, 1982). To create a poem is to rehearse the faculties needed to create the rest of our life. The order and structure of a poem and the ritual of the session can allow the confused mind to achieve clarity, even if only briefly.

Systems/Metacommunication School

This orientation sees the individual as part of a social fabric, interconnected with others and the environment. Changing one part of that fabric will inevitably affect how clients see themselves. Directives, paradox, ritual, and hypnotic phenomena are part of the therapist's armamentarium (Haley, 1973). From this perspective, poetic images possess novelty, complexity, and paradoxicality and embody problems and their solutions. For instance, negative perceptions of women can shift through reframing the story of Eve: "You are the mother of invention / the first scientist. . . . / We are all the children of your bright hunger" (Piercy, 1992, "Applesauce for Eve").

Humanistic/Expressive School

This orientation stresses limitless possibilities for growth and change as individuals actualize their higher being. Techniques include genuine encounter, spontaneity, imagination, evocation of feeling, aliveness in the body, and creativity. Carl Jung (1963) prefigured the therapeutic applications of the arts.

In pure form, any one school of psychotherapy is but a caricature of the complexity of human nature. In practice each in some measure contains all the others. Poetry is multilingual, speaking in the languages of all the psychotherapies. Poems can be found that reveal the unconscious, explore relationships, manifest the clarity of reason, exert indirect influence on behavior, and promote the journey of growth.

POPULATIONS SERVED

In the first 60 issues of the *Journal of Poetry Therapy,* and in the major texts of this form of arts therapy, the interested reader can find articles on poetry therapy across the lifespan: birthing, childhood, adolescence, parenting and adulthood, aging, and dying (Adams, 1990, 2000; Fox, 1995, 1997; Hynes & Hynes-Berry, 1986; Leedy, 1969, 1973; Mazza, 1999; Morrison, 1987; White & Grayson, 1987). Articles addressing gender and diversity and wellness and illness are found in this literature. The literature's clinical spectrum includes alcoholism and other substance abuse, major mental illness, borderline personality disorder, eating disorders (Woodall & Andersen, 1989), surviving sexual abuse, developmental disability, dementia and other brain insults, and HIV/AIDS. Settings discussed include mental hospitals, outpatient clinics, community-based support centers, the mainstream classroom and the special education setting, addiction treatment centers, prisons, nursing homes, and private offices. Individual, group, couple, and family modalities are all represented.

ASSESSMENT

For the most part poetry techniques are not used diagnostically. All persons are potentially capable of responding to the creativity of others with their own creativity. All can be moved and soothed by beauty. All have the capacity to be creators in their own lives, to assume more authority.

Practitioners assess participants' readiness, usually by a trial of therapy. Some few disqualify themselves, but—with suitable adaptations of technique—the range of participants is surprising and includes those recovering from acute psychosis, suffering from dementia, with developmental disability, the undereducated and the illiterate.

Hynes and Hynes-Berry (1986) have devised forms for charting progress, within a session and over time, based on performance rather than pathology.

EDUCATION AND RESEARCH

While the number of courses and workshops given at universities and other venues throughout the country is proliferating, there are not, as of this writing, formal university training programs in poetry therapy—except for students enrolled at schools where they are allowed to customize their studies. Instead, people with a love of literature and a desire to help others grow come from another profession or discipline and train with an approved poetry therapist mentor-supervisor. Those with a psychotherapy degree are eligible to work toward the clinical designation Registered Poetry Therapist. Those from a nonclinical field, such as poets, writers, and teachers, are eligible to work for the developmental designation Certified Poetry Therapist. The training includes didactic study, peer experiential study, and supervised practice.

Writing's salubrious effects on the body in health and illness have been documented (Pennebaker, 1997; Smyth, Stone, Hurewitz, & Kaell, 1999). But despite a growing interest in the use of poetry as a therapeutic modality, there is not a great body of quantitative research in the field of poetry therapy. Mazza (1993) and Hedberg (1997) present a research agenda for the field. Meanwhile, we can take comfort from a robust meta-analysis of the major schools of psychotherapy. It shows that there are no advantages of one form or psychotherapy over another. All are equally effective provided they supply the essential ingredients expected of a professionally trained psychotherapist (Smith, Glass, & Miller, 1980).

THE PROCESS OF POETRY THERAPY

Poetry therapy is an interactive process with three essential components: the poem or some other form of literature, the trained facilitator, and the client(s) (National Coalition of Creative Arts Therapies Associations, 2004). While it is impossible to identify one perfect method for using poetry therapy in treatment, it is possible to describe the most common components used by therapists. Most poetry therapists watch for the "now moment" as an axis of change. While development is continuous, there are critical periods of flowering for successive life tasks, from birth to death (Erikson, 1963).

In a typical session, a therapist selects a poem or other form of imaginal literature to stimulate and evoke feeling responses from the client or clients. This interactive process between the facilitator and the participants helps individuals to experience growth in sensory, emotional, cognitive, intrapersonal, social, and spiritual dimensions in order to enhance their psychological and physical health and well-being.

Criteria for selecting suitable poems include universality, intensity, depth, rhythm, images, metaphors, accessibility of language, clarity of idea, honesty, tone, power of language, openness, and relevance of subject. Mystery, ambiguity, and paradox may be very useful at times. The therapist should be aware of transference/countertransference factors in the selection process (Rolfs & Super, 1988). Effective literature is not abstruse, is culturally sensitive, finds hope in the human condition, is life-affirming, and presents possible solutions without being prescriptive.

The therapist establishes a safe and nonthreatening atmosphere to promote sharing feelings openly and honestly. The first therapeutic task is to welcome, invite, and affirm. Warm-ups for this initial stage may include visualizations or other relaxation techniques, or a very brief statement of feeling-in-the-moment. He or she then introduces the literature, based on participant and group needs. Sometimes *realia*—for example, a stone, seashell, leaf, or household object—is used to illustrate the literature. Other arts media may be used adjunctively. The therapist, or the clients, read the poem aloud, as though it were a story. Giving voice is important; it is a way of embodying the literature. Receptive listening is also important.

Expressive writing techniques may follow. Writing concretizes the elusive. Through writing, the client takes a stand. The therapist tries to put participants at ease about writing: talent is unimportant; the only goal is a genuine response. Many entry techniques for writing can be used (see, e.g., Adams, 1990; Fox, 1995, 1997; Rico, 1983). The poem title, or circled key words, can serve as a takeoff point. The poem can serve as a template, with spaces left blank for clients to fill in. As they become more comfortable, their writing should become freer and more personal. In the sharing period participants may pass, edit, or share fully, depending on their needs for privacy and security.

A poetry therapy session evolves over four stages (Hynes & Hynes-Berry, 1986; National Coalition of Creative Arts Therapies Associations, 2004):

1. *Recognition.* Time is allowed to quietly absorb the piece. "There is something in the material that engages the participant—piques interest, opens the imagination, stops wandering thoughts . . . arrests attention" (Hynes & Hynes-Berry, 1986, pp. 44–45). The therapist invites response: "What do you first notice?" Group interchange is encouraged. No judgments are made about "right" or "wrong" interpretations.

2. *Examination.* "Examination involves the questions who, what, when, why, how, how much, and wherefore" (Hynes & Hynes-Berry, 1986, p. 49). Clients explore their own reactions—for example, their feelings, images, memories, associations, likes and dislikes. The therapist may ask them to underline or to call out words. The literature—its words, images, tone, or argument—evokes individual responses in each client. The therapist should encourage maximum awareness of thoughts, feelings, images, sense perceptions, attitudes, and emotions.

3. *Juxtaposition.* Participants place their responses and those of other participants side by side. They place contrasting elements in the literature side by side. Taking an opposite point of view can encourage new awareness that may inspire new behaviors, attitudes, or values. Eventually arguments with others and arguments within the individuals emerge. Discussion reveals points of pain, degrees of openness, and amounts of self-protection. Conflict reveals our multiplicities and may lead to synthesis.

4. *Application to the Self.* Finally, the individual is encouraged to apply his or her new knowledge to experiences in the real world. At the end of a session, the therapist helps participants integrate what they have

learned. Clients reflect on what needs to be changed and what needs to stay the same, for now. How did the poem help today? How did the writing help? Where do we go from here? A collaborative poem as an ending can provide a group snapshot. After difficult sessions, the therapist should ask whether anyone is uncomfortable, anxious, or needs additional help, and then address specific problems.

CASE EXAMPLES

Case Example 1

> When someone deeply listens to you
> your bare feet are on the earth
> and a beloved land that seemed distant is now at home within you.
> —JOHN FOX (1995, "When Someone
> Deeply Listens to You," p. 58).

As a poetry therapist I went weekly to an acute ward of an inner-city mental hospital. I walked around the dayroom saying hello and introducing myself: "Each week at this time we have a discussion that is interesting and enjoyable. Please join us." Some patients would walk away. Some would politely decline. Some would pace, responding only to their inner voices. I continued in this way until I recruited six to eight people. Anyone who was willing to attend almost always participated successfully. This was the screening test. An uncomfortable few left. Fewer still needed to be asked to leave because of their poor control.

On this spring day I quickly gathered three women and two men. I briefly introduced the group's purpose: "We are here to enjoy each other's company through listening to one another, and learning from each other's life experience. To begin I would like to start the ball rolling with some words written by a person who had an experience important enough to share with us. Then our own words will take over." I gave each participant a copy of a poem I chose for its relevance, brevity, and accessibility. "Today we begin with the words of Carl Sandburg's poem 'The South Wind Says So' " (Sandburg, 1950, p. 226).

The initial reaction of the group was simple pleasure. Henry said he liked it, and several others nodded, except Mrs. Prince, who looked tense and withdrawn. They liked the phrases "song learnt from the south wind" and "we will get by, we will keep on coming." We spent some time at the level of relaxation and group cohesion, hearing who liked or disliked which images and why. Then Steve took the plunge. He rapidly and excitedly posed three questions, with his own rhythm of speech mirroring the poem's. He speeded up, ended emphatically, and pointed to a member of the group seated beside me: "Do you love Kenny? Do you think that all people should be treated equally, no matter what their color? We have needs, are you willing to help us?"

Steve's exclamations caught everyone off guard. Two members moved to protect me by hushing Steve. But I pointed out that Steve was just "coming along, fixing our hearts over" as the poem says. When I gave this permission, the discussion moved on to a deeper level: how hard it is to be heard, how hard it is to take a risk, how Steve sometimes jumps in and cuts others off, how Kenny is reticent to open up and others are concerned about him. Mrs. Prince shared some of her difficulties with her son, who was just out of prison, and was breaking her heart. Elizabeth shared that she was heartbroken when her child was taken by foster care. They received acknowledgments for their sharing.

The hour has passed quickly. For the closing I invited each member to contribute one sentence on the topic "What do I need to do to get by?" I wrote each line on the board, then read aloud the completed collaborative poem.

I thanked everyone for participating. The group members stated this has been a good meeting, a chance to talk. I closed by saying, "I look forward to seeing here again anyone who will still be in the hospital next week. For those who will be discharged meanwhile, I wish you the best."

Postscript

This case illustrates that with rapid participant turnover, each session must be conducted as a completed whole (Yalom, 1983). The poem I used ("The South Wind Says So"), is tailored to this purpose. It is accessible, is brief, has appealing imagery, and is affirmative and encouraging. The accelerated rhythm of the last lines and the eager Steve meshed perfectly to get the ball rolling. The line "We will get by" is repeated twice, the third time shifting to "we will fix our hearts over, / the south wind says so." Members clearly related to the subtext of the healing heart.

This case also illustrates that health and illness are relative. The "sickest" person has something to offer the "healthiest." Sometimes the "sickest" are survivors of some of life's most wounding experiences processed through the most tightly wired sensibilities. Nonetheless, we are all composed of the same "stuff," and this is reflected in a group's response to poetry.

Case Example 2

> We have all been expelled from the Garden,
> But the ones who suffer most in exile are
> Those who are still permitted to dream of
> Perfection.
> —STANLEY KUNITZ (1985, "Seedcorn and
> Windfall")

I worked individually with Amalia, an artistically gifted woman in her 40s, who was born abroad in wartime, the illegitimate child of an emotionally distant young mother and an anonymous father. At age 3 she was sexually abused by a family friend. That same year her family placed her in a loveless orphanage. She remained there until she emigrated to the United States as a young adult.

She was competent at whatever she did, but never stayed long in one career. Her heart remained asleep—until awakened by an exciting man, who then abandoned her. The lava of despair erupted, leaving her suicidal. She wrote a poem for me: "Dark, emptiness, void are my only experiences. . . . Everything reeks of death, end, finality. . . . I want to die, disappear, evaporate in thin air."

I diagnosed attachment disorder and posttraumatic stress disorder. Since Amalia was an avid reader, I suggested and lent books to her as transitional objects. The Scheherezade story from the *Arabian Nights* provided a frame: as long as the next chapter was left open, Amalia's life would go on.

My first absence brought Amalia to the brink of suicide. She left me a phone message that she was about to take her life. I returned her call and read Amalia a poem I composed for this occasion. It referred to mythological figures she would know from her own culture: Persephone, saved by her mother and required to live half the year in this world, half the year in the underworld. My therapeutic poem enjoined: "With the cunning of Ulysses go to the edge of terror / go as far as necessary / but no further / . . . . Remember the future / Remember me as I remember you." Eventually she wrote her response: "In the arid Arab night / the fires sparkles / . . . . At the horizon / sky and land meet / The stars extend their fingers / to be kissed by the fire." I also wrote for myself a countertransference poem, in anticipatory grief, and as a magic to prevent a suicidal disaster: "pulling apart / I go my own way / returning to the earth whence I sprang / joyous at last / dancing dust mote held by the tender breeze." Contact was maintained. She survived.

During her next suicidal crisis, I composed a creation myth for her. A Phoenix who has exhausted her regenerative powers is given gifts by the forest creatures who surround her: the ability to hibernate, the skill of burying and locating nuts, the knack of making a home by felling trees, the ability to curl up and dream. The patient wrote in response: "Outside / a group of pine trees give shelter / In the middle / a mound of pine needles / on the mound a ring of muck / white summer mold / Surprise / a live thing that shoots sparks and multiplies / Disgust / an infection that needs to be destroyed." In discussion it became clear to me that feeling alive was scary to Amalia because that feeling of excitement had always heralded the danger of loss and abandonment.

Later Amalia wrote: "Dark wings cover my lifeless form / Roots siphon my life / I have found my home / Next season I will be the tallest tree / The brightest flower / the greenest leaf / The first branch to greet the sun rise / The first to be drenched by the storm / The first to be struck down again."

At another session I offered her a basket of evocative words I had cut from magazines. From "gifts," "repeat," and "hand," she composed: "The Queen of flowers / taking the hand of the girl / said with great love / You have no choice / the gifts are yours / do as you please / Waste / Or use wisely / If you waste / You will have to repeat / the whole story again."

Further along in therapy she wrote: "the air is quite warm and scented with primroses, spring honeysuckle, columbine, wild astelbe, cyclamens, fresh cut grass, sweet hay drying in the sun, moist ground. . . . an intoxicating mixture. . . . I feel internally happy, content, at peace, in equilibrium. Another crisis has been averted. I try to capture the feeling created by nature to reward those that take time to rest with her . . . the coveted reward of satisfied lovers, to immortalize it in my mind and heart."

Postscript

The fine paradox here is that, in order to live, Amalia had to keep herself emotionally dead, and in coming alive she felt she had to die. Her loves of nature and of writing were two attachments to build on. Poetry was not a magic bullet to protect her against suicide. Antidepressants were useful in this situation, and I obtained consultation from suicide experts when agonizing about whether to hospitalize Amalia involuntarily. My recognition of countertransference feelings, aided by my own writing, was a useful tool in helping me to keep emotional balance in the face of those countertransference feelings. Therapists should not routinely offer their own work as the poetic stimulus to clients because writing to, and for, the patient is a highly specific technique that requires special training, experience, and supervision.

Case Example 3

> Anyone who breathes is in the rhythm business;
> anyone who is alive is caught up in the imminces,
> the doubts mixed with the triumphant uncertainty
> of poetry.
> —WILLIAM STAFFORD

"I never expected this, but what else can it be now?," Louise said resignedly to her fellow members of the retirement community's widows/widowers group.

Her stooped posture and lined face reflected the disasters of the last 3 of her 77 years. But her matching bracelet and pin suggested that she was a tasteful woman who still took pride in her appearance.

First, Nathan, her mate of 46 years, her constant companion and playmate, her lord and master, had dropped dead on the golf course, joining too many of her friends and relatives at Morningside Cemetery. Then her own heart condition worsened, cutting her energy reserves. And now her two children, living at a distance, had insisted that she give up her beloved home and move into a one-bedroom apartment in the euphemistically named Sunrise Heights. To her, it looked all downhill from here.

As Louise looked around the circle, three or four faces familiar to her from the dining room nodded in greeting. Her companions here ranged in age from 68 to 89, and their health was variable. Two men stared down the floor, making no effort. Two women exchanged animated whispers. She counted one cane, two walkers, and an ugly wheelchair among her eight companions, and wondered to herself how soon she would need one of these "appliances," so unlike the shiny machines she had chosen for her first household.

I welcomed the participants to this first meeting, inviting them to share their voices, imaginations, life experiences, and creative abilities. I distributed copies of "How to Eat a Poem" (Merriam, 1967), asking participants to keep it face down. As a warm-up, I invited members to savor a small cup of orange juice, noting its color, temperature, and flavor, and their own reactions. Each person around the circle gave his or her name and his or her reaction to the juice. I read the poem, then asked volunteers to read it again, after ascertaining that everyone could read and hear well enough. This poem gives permission: "Don't be polite / Bite in / . . . You do not need / . . . napkin or tablecloth. . . . " I asked, "What are your reactions to the idea that in this group we don't have to maintain polite formalities, we can get personal and be spontaneous?" Louise said she did not like the idea of the juice running down her arm—it might ruin a good blouse.

Next I offered "Jeronimo's House" (Bishop, 1983), lovingly described as "my perishable clapboard fairy palace," with its "center table / of woven wicker / painted blue / . . . an old French horn / . . . I play each year in the parade / for Jose Marti / . . . my radio/singing flamencos / . . . When I move / I take these things / not much more, from / my shelter from / the hurricane." Louise begged off from reading the poem, saying "I don't have enough breath today," even though she was not short of breath when she walked into the room or helped to arrange the chairs. I chose to honor her request, in exchange for a promise to "lend us your voice" another time. In ensuing weeks, Louise's voice did grow stronger.

Following this poem, I asked participants to list in one column things they had to leave behind when they moved here, and in another column the things they had brought with them. Everyone told of mixed feelings about closing their last household. Then for 5 minutes they wrote about one possession they had to abandon, and one they selected to accompany them. After sharing and discussion, the group ended with a collaborative poem, with each person calling out one line from what he or she had written. This engendered lively interest as I wrote the lines on the whiteboard. Louise wrote about the old Singer sewing machine she had inherited from her mother that, happily, her own daughter had taken. Both love to sew.

The second session began with "names." The poem "Signing My Name" (Townsend, 1996) launched the discussion. The speaker in the poem recalls how her mother had taught her, at age 6, to sign her name to her art work: "She dipped the brush for me / and watched while I stroked my name / each letter drying ruddy / permanent as blood."

I asked the participants, "How did you get your name? What nicknames were you called, and how did you feel about them? How would you like to be addressed here? What name would you give yourself in this moment?" Members then shared their childhood memories around names. Louise was named for her mother's favorite sister, who became her favorite aunt, and was a warm, fun-loving person. Louise smiled when she disclosed that her girlfriends called her "Beeney Louie," skinny as a stringbean: "I wish I had that svelte appearance now, instead of all these extra pounds."

I directed participants to block-letter their first name down the left side of a blank page. I asked them to "describe yourself, beginning each line with each successive letter in your name." Louise shared: "Living each day is uncertain / Only yesterday I was a young wife / Until Nathan died I thought my life was full / Instants of good times flash through my mind / Seldom do I feel happy now / Everyday I hope will be better." The group acknowledged Louise's grief, and several other members shared their feelings and thoughts about death. There was agreement to pursue this important subject in subsequent meetings.

The next several weeks were spent discussing deaths of loved ones. Grieving would never be over. It would come in waves of greater or lesser sharpness, and it would always hover. Participants were learning to live with it. From talk about the deaths of parents, siblings, spouses, and friends, the conversation shifted to talk about one's own mortality: illnesses, disabilities, disappointments, fears, loss of dreams. One of the poems that helped during this time asked: "Body my house / my horse my hound / what will I do / when you are fallen / Where will I sleep / How will I ride . . . ?" (Swenson, 2000, "Question," p. 882). I asked participants to circle key words or phrases "that jump out at you." Louise circled "body my house," "danger or treasure," "how will I hide?" All members did likewise, wrote their own poems using the keywords, and shared. Louise wrote: "How can I trust you, old friend? Still, let us help one another."

This opened the door to discussion of feelings about death, burial plans, wills, and legacies. Three members said they would initiate discussion with their doctors and children to document their living will and health care proxy. Members discussed fear of pain, of incapacity, of abandonment. Two members expressed a desire to spare their children the final deterioration; the others, Louise among them, wanted their children and grandchildren to gather for a final blessing. Louise noted that after this blessing, she would like to be left alone with her daughter until the end. The idea arose to dispense more of those blessings right now, during family visits and outings. There was a brief discussion about belief, or nonbelief, in an afterlife. After Pete said, "I sure wish I could attend my own funeral to hear what people are going to say about me," we agreed to focus on eulogies at the next session.

In the eulogy session, Louise wrote: "Louise was strong though quiet. She built her life around her love for her husband and children. She was a shelter and tower of strength and it filled her. She cooked with love, went to her sons' games with love, taught her daughter to sew and tended her garden with love." Love entered the group. Members shared appreciations and supportive comments with one another. Louise reaped a great deal of appreciation. She glowed.

Group liveliness increased during the next few weeks. "The Round" (Kunitz, 1995) was written at age 80 by a poet who, at age 95, when asked when his next book would be published, answered, "Be patient, I'm working on it." "Light splashed this morning / on the shell-pink anemones / . . . I can scarcely wait till tomorrow / when a new life begins for me / as it does each day / as it does each day." Members recalled for one another the beautiful moments, not unmixed with sorrows and anxieties, of their lives today. Louise lit up at someone's use of the phrase "late bloomers." "Why that's what I've been doing these last few months, enjoying my art classes, leading the prayer group, and making a scrapbook of my life, putting that old boxful of pictures to good use, really drinking in pleasure from family visits." I then asked, "What does the 'compost heap' in this poem mean to the group?" Louise responded, "I have learned that making mistakes is OK. Stop trying to be so perfect. Mistake is just another name for learning. Now mistakes are my compost heap."

Postscript

Sometimes we pigeonhole older people into reminiscence groups, forgetting that they are still alive and still have the capacity to grow. Louise learned to be alone, to get past some of the limits of neatness, niceness, and perfectionism. She, and others, felt relief and release discussing their final wishes.

CAUTIONS IN USING POEMS IN THERAPY

As seen in the case examples, literature is a power tool. But therapists must remember it can harm as well as heal if not used skillfully (Lauer, 1994; Pies, 1993). The movie *Dead Poets Society* depicts a teen who commits suicide when he is trapped between feelings of freedom aroused by a charismatic teacher and the rigid repression of his father. In a real situation, a 12-year-old returned from school in tears. During Black History Month, an artist-in-the-schools had brought in and played a Billie Holiday recording of "Strange Fruit." It contained graphic images of a lynching. The artist read the lyrics, played the song, and then spoke briefly about the history of segregation and the black experience. She moved to a different topic, leaving a huge emotional charge in the kids. Unfortunately she was not attuned to issues of safety, timing, context, chance to process feelings, maturational age, and so on. The artist did not ask herself, "What is the goal here? What methods are suitable or unsuitable?" In all likelihood, the artist had not checked in with her countertransference feelings and had not considered the powerful impact words can have in seemingly benign situations.

CONCLUSION

The word/was born in the blood
grew in the dark body, beating
and flew through the lips and the mouth.
—PABLO NERUDA, (1970, "The Word," p. 431).

Poetry therapy is, along with drama therapy, the newest of the organized creative arts therapies and expressive therapies. Like these therapies, its roots go back to the beginnings of humankind. Today's profession is eclectic in membership and in theoretical orientation. Poetry therapy has been applied across a broad spectrum of developmental, clinical, and mind–body applications.

Poetry is a mirror, a disguise, a bridge. Poetry is continuity, it is change. It is large in its smallness. It embraces and transcends conflict; it is both/and rather than either/or. Poetry is individual and communal. It is thought and action. Its wordplay makes masks and penetrates disguises and invites intimacy ("into-me-see").

REFERENCES

Adams, K. (1990). *Journal to the self.* New York: Warner Books.
Adams, K. (2000). *The write way to wellness.* Lakewood, CO: Center for Journal Therapy.

Alexander, A., & French, T. (1974). *Psychoanalytic therapy: Principles and application.* Lincoln: University of Nebraska Press.

Bettelheim, B. (1977). *The uses of enchantment: The meaning and importance of fairy tales.* New York: Vintage Books.

Bishop, E. (1983). Jeronimo's house. In *The complete poems of Elizabeth Bishop, 1927–1979* (p. 34). New York: Farrar, Straus & Giroux.

Christensen, P. (1986). Magical properties of the poem. In M. Morrison (Ed.), *Poetry as therapy* (pp. 87–99). New York: Human Sciences Press.

Cox, M., & Theilgaard, A. (1986). *Mutative metaphors in psychotherapy: The Aolian mode.* New York: Tavistock.

Erikson, E. H. (1963). *Childhood and society.* New York: Norton.

Fox, J. (1995). *Finding what you didn't lose.* New York: Tarcher/Putnam.

Fox, J. (1997). *Poetic medicine: The healing art of poem-making.* New York: Tarcher/Putnam.

Goldfried, M., & Newman, C. (1986). Psychotherapy integration: An historical perspective. In J. Norcross (Ed.), *Handbook of eclectic psychotherapy* (pp. 25–60). New York: Brunner/Mazel.

Gorelick, K. (1987). Greek tragedy and ancient healing: Poems as theatre and Aesculepian temple in miniature. *Journal of Poetry Therapy, 1*(1), 38–43.

Gorelick, K. (1989). Rapprochement between the arts and psychotherapies. *Arts in Psychotherapy, 16,* 149–155.

Haley, J. (1973). *The uncommon therapy: The psychiatric techniques of Milton Erikson.* New York: Norton.

Hedberg, T. M. (1997). The re-enchantment of poetry therapy. *International Journal of the Arts in Psychotherapy, 24*(1), 91–100.

Heller, P. O. (1995). *Poetry therapy training manual for mental health professionals.* Unpublished doctoral dissertation, Pacific Western University.

Hynes, A., & Hynes-Berry, M. (1986). *Bibliotherapy the interactive process: A handbook.* St. Cloud, MN: North Star Press.

Johnson, D. R. (1999). Refining the developmental paradigm in the creative arts therapies. In *Essays on the creative arts therapies* (pp. 161–181). Springfield, IL: Thomas.

Jung, C. G. (1963). *Memories, dreams and reflections.* New York: Basic Books.

Kuhl, P. (2002). Language, rain and mind: Early experience alters the perception of speech. *Irvine Health Foundation Lectures.* Available online at *www.ihf.org/lecture/archive/kuhl.html.*

Kunitz, S. (1985). Seedcorn and windfall. In *Next-to-last things.* Boston: Atlantic Monthly Press.

Kunitz, S. (1995). The round. In *Passing through* (pp. 128–129). New York: Norton.

Lauer, R. (1994). Abuses of poetry therapy. In A. Lerner (Ed.), *Poetry in the therapeutic experience* (2nd ed., pp. 73–80). St. Louis, MO: MMB Music.

Leedy, J. J. (Ed.). (1969). *Poetry therapy: The use of poetry in the treatment of emotional disorders.* Philadelphia: Lippincott.

Leedy, J. J. (Ed.). (1973). *Poetry the healer.* Philadelphia: Lippincott.

Lerner, A. (Ed.). (1994). *Poetry in the therapeutic experience*. St. Louis, MO: MMB Music.

Lux, T. (1997). *New and selected poems, 1975–1995*. New York: Houghton Mifflin.

Mazza, N. (1993). Poetry therapy: Toward a research agenda for the 1990's. *International Journal for the Arts in Psychotherapy, 20*(1), 51–59.

Mazza, N. (1999). *Poetry therapy: Interface of the arts and psychology*. Boca Raton, FL: CRC Press.

Merriam, E. (1967). How to eat a poem. In S. Dunning et al. (Eds.), *Reflections on a gift of watermelon pickle*. New York: Lothrop, Lee and Shepard.

Morrison, M. R. (1982). *A historic review of the use of poetry in psychotherapy from archaic ritual to ancient therapeutic practice: Toward a theory of poetry therapy*. Unpublished doctoral dissertation, University for Humanistic Studies, San Diego, CA.

Morrison, M. R. (1987). *Poetry as therapy*. New York: Human Sciences Press.

National Coalition of Creative Arts Therapies Associations. (2004). Poetry therapy. Available online at *www.nccata.org/poetry.html/*.

Neruda, P. (1970). The word. In N. Tarn (Ed.), *Pablo Neruda: Selected poems*. New York: Houghton Mifflin.

Oliver, M. (1983). In blackwater woods. In *American primitive* (pp. 82–83). Boston: Little Brown.

Pennebaker, J. (1997). *Opening up*. New York: Guilford Press.

Pies, R. (1993). Adverse reaction to poetry therapy: A case study report. *Journal of Poetry Therapy, 6*(3), 143–147.

Piercy, M. (1992). Applesauce for Eve. In *Mars and her children*. New York: Knopf.

Reiter, S. (2004). A brief overview of poetry therapy. In *Guide to training requirements for trainers and trainees for certification and registration as a poetry therapist* (pp. 1–4). Washington, DC: National Federation for Biblio/Poetry.

Rico, G. (1983). *Writing the natural way*. New York: Tarcher/Putnam.

Rolfs, A., & Super, S. (1988). Guiding the unconscious: The process of poem selection for poetry therapy groups. *Arts in Psychotherapy, 15*, 119–126.

Sandburg, S. (1950). *Complete poems*. New York: Harcourt Brace.

Shrodes, C. (1960). Bibliotherapy: An application of psychoanalytical theory. *American Image, 17*, 311–319.

Smith, M., Glass, G., & Miller, T. (1980). *The benefits of psychotherapy*. Baltimore: Johns Hopkins University Press.

Smyth, J., Stone, A., Hurewitz, A., & Kaell, A. (1999). Effects of writing about stressful experiences on symptom reduction in patients with asthma or rheumatoid arthritis. *Journal of the American Medical Association, 281*(14), 1304–1309.

Swenson, M. (2000). Question. In *American poetry: The twentieth century* (Vol. 2, p. 882). New York: The Library of America.

Taylor, C. B. (1982). Treatment evaluation and behavior therapy. In M. Lewis & G.

Usdin (Eds.), *Treatment planning in psychiatry* (pp. 151–224). Washington, DC: American Psychiatric Association.

Townsend, A. (1996). Signing my name. In M. Sewell (Ed.), *Claiming the spirit within* (p. 197). Boston: Beacon Press.

White, A., & Grayson, D. (1987). *Parents and other strangers.* New York: Ashley Books.

Woodall, C., & Andersen, A. E. (1989). The use of metaphor and poetry therapy in the treatment of the reticent subgroup of anorectic patients. In L. M. Hornyak & E. K. Baker (Eds.), *Experiential therapies for eating disorders* (pp. 191–206). New York: Guilford Press.

Woolridge, S. (1996). *Poemcrazy.* New York: Three Rivers Press.

Yalom, I. (1970). *The theory and practice of group psychotherapy.* New York: Basic Books.

Yalom, I. (1983). *Inpatient group psychotherapy.* New York: Basic Books.

Play Therapy

LINDA E. HOMEYER
EMILY DEFRANCE

HISTORY

Play therapy, a specific form of child psychotherapy, is nearly as old as psychotherapy itself. The name of Freud, only this time Anna, shows up among the first play therapists. Anna, like so many who followed her, knew the importance of providing mental health services for children. These early play therapists also knew the impact of human development on the ability to provide such services.

Play is the environment and experience within which children learn about their world and their experiences in that world. Haim Ginott (1961) coined the phrase "The child's play is his talk and the toys are his words." Using toys, the materials with which they feel comfortable, children are able to express that for which they do not have the words. This inability to use words may be based in their cognitive developmental level, their fear of their own safety if the family secret becomes known, or their inability to face the overwhelming and incapacitating emotional and psychological power of their life experience. Toys provide a symbolic expression when they as yet do not have the symbols of words. Toys provide a way to "show" what has happened when they have been threatened not to "tell." Toys provide the emotional and psychological distancing to allow communication while containing their own over-whelming emotions. Toys are indeed the words, and play the language.

While Anna Freud (1965) and Melanie Klein (1932) were develop-ing the psychoanalytic approach to play therapy, Margaret Lowenfeld (1993) was also developing a method of working with children by using play. Dr. Lowenfeld, who spoke several languages, found it difficult to put into words her work with refugee families during the Russo–Polish War. As she sought some nonverbal way in which children could express their experiences, she remembered a book she had read many years prior, *Floor Games*, by H. G. Wells (1911). In this book, Wells describes lengthy, elaborate stories he played out with his two sons on the floor of a room in their home using a variety of miniature toys. With this creative play in mind, Lowenfeld developed her World Technique through which "direct contact could be made, without interference from the adult, with the mental and emotional life of a child" (p. 3). Jungian analyst Dora Kalff modified Lowenfeld's technique by encouraging children to "make a world" in a tray filled one-third with sand (Allan & Berry, 1987; Carey, 1999; DeDomenico, 1994; Homeyer & Sweeney, 1998; Hunter, 1998; Kalff, 1971, 1980; Oaklander, 1988).

The first shift in play therapy was to a directed format within the psychoanalytic framework. David Levy (1933, 1939) in release play therapy, Gove Hambidge (1955) in structured play therapy, and J. Solo-mon (1938) in active play therapy used specific toys to help children set up scenarios to work through specific issues. These approaches were pri-marily developed to work with children who lived in an overall healthy home situation but who were not able to adjust adequately to a particu-lar stressful life event.

The next major movement in play therapy continued to mirror the changes in the broad field of psychotherapy. Virginia Axline (1969) de-veloped nondirective play therapy. Her work was an application of Carl Rogers's client-centered therapy (1951). Her classic case study, *Dibs* (1971), remains one of the best-selling books in the field of child psycho-therapy. Louise Guerney (1969, 1992) and Garry Landreth (1991) are major influences in this area, now generally called child-centered play therapy (Landreth & Sweeney, 1997).

Other humanistic-oriented play therapists also valued the impor-tance of the relationship between the child and the therapist and conse-quently developed relationship play therapy. Clark Moustakas (1953, 1966, 1992), who drew upon the work of Jesse Taft and Otto Rank, was the leading proponent of this type of play therapy. Carol Norton and Byron Norton (1997), heavily influenced by Moustakas, have written about experiential play therapy, a further outgrowth of the humanistic approach.

At about this same time, developmental play therapy was created by Viola Brody (1993). Her work focused on the interaction, or dialogue, between the therapist and the child through the use of playful touch. This form of play therapy is especially appropriate for children with disruptions in attachment and bonding. Ann Jernberg (1979) developed her own form of this play therapy, which she named Theraplay.

As the field continued to grow and develop, psychodynamic theories of counseling were applied to play therapy. John Allan wrote extensively on Jungian play therapy (Allan, 1988, 1997; Allan & Bertoia, 1992; Allan & Brown, 1993). Judi Bertoia (1999) and J. P. Lilly (2003) continue to write and practice in this area. Violet Oaklander (1988), a Gestalt child therapist, uses many expressive arts with children including art, sandtray, and play therapy. Adlerian play therapy, based on Adler's individual psychology, was developed by Terry Kottman (1987, 1995, 1999; Kottman & Johnson, 1993; Kottman & Stiles, 1990; Kottman & Warlick, 1989, 1990).

The cognitive-behavioral forces in psychotherapy were felt in the play therapy field as well. *Cognitive-Behavioral Play Therapy*, written by Susan Knell (1993), reflects this directive method of working with children. The play therapist diagnoses the issue that needs treatment and then develops structured play to use with the child to resolve that issue.

Two recent approaches to play therapy are the ecosystemic and the prescriptive. Ecosystemic play therapy is an integrative approach developed by Kevin O'Connor (1991, 2000; O'Connor & Ammen, 1997). It is a comprehensive developmental and systemic approach. The play therapist is to be very aware of the many systems affecting the client's functioning. These include socioeconomic, ethnic, cultural, legal, family, school, peers, religion, and social services (O'Connor, 2000). A special strength of O'Connor's approach is his stress on the assessment of developmental levels, particularly cognition, behavior, communication, and socialization. O'Connor states that "the play therapist has a primary role in developing and implementing a treatment plan that will maximize the client's developmental functioning while minimizing her symptomatology" (2000, p. 204).

Heidi Kaduson, Donna Cangelosi, and Charles Schaefer (1997) developed prescriptive play therapy. In this application of play therapy, the play therapist diagnoses the problem and matches, or prescribes, the play therapy techniques or theoretical approach to fit the needs of the child client.

MAJOR THEORETICAL ORIENTATIONS

As the previous section delineates, there are many play therapy theories, all with passionate adherents and anecdotal research that support the theory that each is successful with most children. A helpful distinction to make when conceptualizing the range of play therapy theories is that between *nondirective* and *directive* approaches. These can be arranged on a continuum, with various theories occupying certain positions on a "directiveness of the therapist" continuum (see Figure 7.1). As Virginia Axline (1947), who was the major developer of child-centered play therapy (then called "nondirective play therapy"), explained, "Play therapy may be directive in form—that is, the therapist may assume responsibility for guidance and interpretation, or it may be nondirective; the therapist may leave responsibility and direction to the child" (p. 9).

The three theories that we have chosen to explore are based on a consensus of leading play therapists: Child-Centered, Adlerian, and Jungian. These three theoretical orientations may be those most valuing the use of the expressive arts by today's practitioners of play therapy.

Child-Centered Play Therapy

Child-centered play therapy is, of course, at the nondirective extreme of the continuum. Its focus is on the child as the source of his or her own

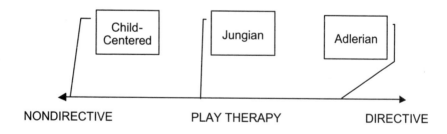

FIGURE 7.1. Nondirective directive continuum.

positive growth and therapeutic direction, fostered by the therapist who provides the "good growing ground" described by Axline (1947, p. 10)—the appropriate climate for the child to experience self fully and to experience his or her own potential for growth (Perry, 1993). This "good growing ground" is the therapeutic relationship in which the child feels secure and safe enough to experience his or her entire emotional range, which may have been kept from his or her awareness as either too threatening or too incongruent with his or her own conditional sense of self.

The child-centered therapeutic relationship is based on Axline's (1947, pp. 66–67) eight basic principles. The therapist must:

1. Develop a warm, friendly relationship with the child.
2. Accept each child exactly as he or she is, without wanting to change the child in any way.
3. Maintain an accepting environment where the child feels free to express all emotions.
4. Recognize and acknowledge the child's feelings in a manner that helps the child gain insight into his or her behavior.
5. Demonstrate a deep and abiding respect for the child's ability to solve his or her own problems, allowing the responsibility for choices and change to be the child's.
6. Make no attempts to direct the child's play or verbal expression; allow the child to lead in all things.
7. Do not hurry the therapeutic process; again, follow the child's lead.
8. Establish only those limits necessary to meet safety, legal, and ethical standards.

"Techniques" of the child-centered play therapist consist of those behaviors that facilitate the "good growing ground" of therapy. The therapist provides *facilitative responses*, including the reflection of content and feeling, to communicate to the child that the therapist is there for the child and is maximally involved in the play therapy experience. He or she also may ask questions to clarify the reality of the child's experience, but refuses to use questions to further the therapist's hypotheses or to satisfy his or her own curiosity about the child. Rather, questions are perceived to be intrusive and as attempts to direct the experience with the child. A second "technique" is that of *structuring* the therapy, to provide a certain rather limited amount of information for the child about the logistics of the therapy, so that the child will know what to expect from the therapist about the length of sessions, where the sessions will occur, whether the parents will be involved and how, and so on. Further structuring responses will be offered in relation to the child's questions about specific activities, always couched in terms that return responsibility to the child ("In here, you can decide").

A third important "technique" involves the setting of limits to allow the child to define for him- or herself the areas in which he or she is free to operate; to allow the therapist to remain empathic and accepting of the child; to ensure the safety of the child, the therapist, and the play environment; and to help the child develop self-control. The focus is on the process of setting the limit within the relationship in a way that enhances the therapeutic encounter. Landreth (1991) has outlined the process in limit setting:

A—Acknowledge the child's feelings, wishes, wants, and behavior ("I see that you are angry and would like to hit me");

C—Communicate the limit broken by the behavior ("But I am not for hitting");

T—Target acceptable behavioral alternatives ("The Bobo is for hitting, or you can pretend that that doll is me and hit it if you choose").

Limits are kept to a minimum, addressed only when needed, and are kept "predictable and consistent as a brick wall" (Guerney, 1983, p. 39). Landreth's (1991) "ultimate limit," used if the child breaks the limit, is to set the consequence ("If you choose to hit me, then you choose not to play any more today," or "If you choose to throw the sand out of the sandbox, then you choose not to play with the sand anymore today") and then to follow through with it.

Toys are seen as the child's words, and play as the child's communication, so the toys in the playroom are specifically chosen to maximize the child's choice of expression. Landreth (1991) cites three categories of toys that facilitate the child's communication: real-life, acting-out and aggressive-release, and creative-expressive and emotional-release toys. Abundant expressive arts materials are displayed in the playroom for children to use as they are drawn to these forms of expression. All the toys and materials are consistently available in the playroom so that the child returns each time to the same environment. The playroom is only cleaned up by the therapist after the child leaves to be sure that the child continues to feel that his or her play (communication) is valued and respected, and not something to be "cleaned up" or undone.

The provision of these essential therapeutic conditions allows the child to fully experience all parts of self and his or her life experiences, to be able to move toward self-actualization.

Adlerian Play Therapy

Another theoretical model of play therapy is Adlerian play therapy, which is more at the directive side of the continuum (although not the most directive form of play therapy, by any means). During the first stage of Adlerian play therapy, many nondirective techniques are used to develop the relationship between the child and the therapist. This approach was developed by Terry Kottman as an integration of the concepts and strategies of individual psychology developed by Alfred Adler, with the rationale, materials, and techniques of play therapy (Kottman, 1993, 1995, 2001). Those principles of Adlerian therapy that provide the grounding for Adlerian play therapy include the following (Kottman, 1994, p. 5):

- Children are inherently social beings who have a need to belong, and each child examines his or her own family to decide how best to fit in.
- Children's behavior is purposeful and goal-oriented, and children are drawn toward the goals of believing they are capable, that they count, that they connect with others in meaningful ways, and that they have enough courage to accomplish life's tasks.
- Children are creative and unique, and are capable of making choices to facilitate movement toward the attainment of their goals.
- Children experience life from a subjective perspective, and the therapist attempts to understand the child's phenomenological experience to in turn help the child begin to understand his or her goals and to be able to achieve them in more constructive, self-affirming, and satisfying ways.

Maladjustment is seen as a form of discouragement, based on the child's inability to find useful, satisfying ways of belonging and feeling significant in his or her life. Such children have developed negative, maladaptive beliefs about themselves, others, and the world, and their self-defeating, sometimes self-destructive goals, behaviors, and attitudes reflect these mistaken convictions.

The goals of intervention in Adlerian play therapy (Kottman, 1997, p. 315) are to help the child:

- Gain an awareness of and insight into his or her lifestyle, formed from experiences within his or her family of origin.
- Alter faulty, self-defeating perceptions of self, others, and the world and move from these faulty convictions (private logic) to common sense.
- Move toward positive goals of behavior.
- Replace negative strategies for belonging and gaining significance with positive, constructive strategies.
- Increase his or her social interest and sense of belonging.
- Learn new ways of coping with life's disappointments, rather than becoming discouraged.
- Optimize his or her creativity to use his or her own assets to develop self-enhancing, rather than self-defeating, choices about his or her attitudes, feelings, and behaviors.

Adlerian play therapy takes place in four nonlinear overlapping phases, each containing its own strategies and techniques. The first phase of therapy is *building an egalitarian, caring relationship between child and therapist,* in which both have choices and both have limits. Some of the techniques used in this phase are nondirective ones such as tracking the child's behavior, restating content, and reflecting feelings; giving explanations and answering the child's questions as needed; asking questions about the child's perceptions about coming to therapy; and structuring the therapy to provide information about logistics, cleaning the playroom together, and setting limits. Adlerian play therapists actively involve parents and teachers (when appropriate) in the therapy; in this first phase, the primary intervention is to listen to the parent(s) empathically and to encourage any positive aspect of their parenting.

In the second phase of Adlerian play therapy, *assessment,* the therapist gathers information about the child's lifestyle (the child's personal orientation to life, his or her plan for gaining significance) from many sources. These include interviews of the child, parents, and teachers; observations of the child's interactions with these important people in his or her life; and various assessment activities within the play sessions (such as having the child complete the Kinetic Family Drawing; make a body outline and discuss the child's sense of self; having the child describe his or her family using dollhouse figures or puppets; eliciting early recollections; exploring the child's behavioral goals; and using questioning strategies). Expressive arts materials are seen to be crucial in this assessment phase of the therapy in gathering lifestyle information. The therapist uses this information to formulate hypotheses about the child's means of gaining significance; his or her self-defeating convictions about self, others, and the world; and other elements of the lifestyle.

In this second phase, the therapist also uses questioning strategies with the parents to attempt to understand their perception of their child and their own lifestyles. Moreover, the therapist attempts to evaluate the impact of the parents' personal priorities (their own personal issues and goals) on their ability to apply parenting skills. Some beginning teaching of parenting skills may also occur in this phase.

The third phase of therapy, *helping the child and the parents to gain insight into the child's lifestyle*, allows parents to understand where the child is coming from, and enables the child to make choices about how to best get his or her needs met. The therapist tentatively shares inferences about the child's goals of behavior, his or her faulty convictions, and how he or she gains significance in the family and at school. The therapist uses interpretations of the child's verbalizations and play and metacommunicates to the child about patterns in his or her behavior that limit his or her ability to get his or her needs met. "By using the child's metaphors, designing therapeutic metaphors, and telling one another stories, the therapist capitalizes on the element of play as the key factor in the child's communication" (Kottman, 1997, p. 329). Extensive use of expressive arts materials is made in helping the child develop insight into his or her lifestyle, whether or not his or her goals are being met, and in deciding whether to change his or her behaviors toward meeting those goals. During this phase too the therapist attempts to make connections between what happens in the playroom and the child's interactions outside the playroom.

The fourth phase of therapy, *reorientation/reeducation*, is designed to help the child learn skills for developing alternative behaviors, and then practicing them so that he or she can use them successfully outside the therapeutic environment. Some of these skills include problem solving, generating alternative behaviors for problematic situations, learning more socially appropriate behaviors, developing better communication skills, and learning negotiating skills. These are at first practiced in the playroom using role play with puppets, dollhouse figures, sandtray, and psychodrama, and are then generalized to specific activities in the real world outside the playroom. The therapist works with the parents to use their new parenting skills consistently, and to develop new perceptions about their child and his or her needs and behaviors. In all four phases, liberal use of encouragement enhances the child's and the parents' abilities to face their discouragement and learn new, more satisfying ways of meeting their various life goals.

Jungian Play Therapy

Jungian play therapy is not a mainstream approach, but it lends itself well to the expressive arts, so we have included it here. It is perhaps midway on our nondirective—directive continuum, as it involves components of both types of approaches.

This model of play therapy is based on the psychological theory of Carl G. Jung's analytical psychology. While Jung did not work directly with children, several subsequent Jungians developed therapeutic strategies for working with children, beginning with Dora Kalff's development of sandplay (which is discussed more fully in Chapter 8 in this volume). John Allan (1988) and his students may have been the first Jungian therapists to directly modify Jungian theory for use with children, both in play therapy and in terms of using it in school counseling, both individually and in groups.

Although analytical psychology is a very complex system, several Jungian concepts are relevant for this discussion of its application to play therapy. Jung believed that the *psyche*, the totality of human subjective experience, was activated by pure life energy (*libido*), fueled by the tension between opposites, such as good and bad, male and female, birth and death, light and dark, and the like. The psyche is made up of three parts:

1. The *ego* is an individual's conscious awareness of the sum total of his or her experiences with him- or herself and the world. It is the center of consciousness and mediates between the demands of the inner world (personal and collective unconscious) and the demands of the outer world (reality).
2. The *personal unconscious* is the repository of material that is both suppressed and repressed, too painful or threatening for the ego to deal with, as well as untapped, undeveloped potentials of the personality.

3. Below the personal unconscious is the *collective unconscious*, which is the "wired-in" connection we all possess with our ancestral past from the beginning of human history, and which contains the archetypes.

Archetypes are instincts coupled with images that direct and influence our emotions and behavior. Archetypes are found universally in art, folklore and myths, and religious expression, and bring an experience of psychological kinship to each individual with others with which we share this planet. They center around the core images of birth, death, love, the Great Mother, the Wise Old Man, the Divine Child, God, the Devil, and so on. Bertoia (1999) characterizes the world of archetypes as a kind of "inner village," with the various archetypes closer to or farther from the individual's conscious accessibility. "Thus, by virtue of being human, everyone's 'village'—their collective unconscious—has the archetypal potential for a divine child and a Hitler, an evil witch and a Mother Teresa" (Bertoia, 1999, p. 88). The archetype of the Self is the central organizing principle of the psyche, out of which the personality develops.

At birth, the ego is embedded in the archetype of the Self (in the unconscious). The ego develops during infancy and early childhood by a process of deintegration and reintegration. That is, the fledgling ego shatters under the normal pressures of hunger, pain, and so on, and reintegrates when comfort is provided. Thus, an important component of the process of reintegration is how well the infant's caregiver(s) mediate the infant's distress and bring about consistent calming and comforting. When this happens well enough and consistently enough, the infant introjects positive images of the mother/father, associated with feelings of comfort and relief, and bonding occurs. As this continues happening, the child develops more and more effective coping skills and ego defenses. If, however, the deintegration process is not met with this interpersonal calming and comforting, then negative images of the parents are introjected, leaving the child believing that his or her very life is in danger. Emotionally wounded children are therefore often unaware of their intense painful feelings, cannot cope with them, and the feelings emerge violently and chaotically in acting-out behaviors over which the child has no adequate control.

Two other archetypes are important for understanding personality development. One of the first archetypal structures to form out of the archetype of the Self is the *persona*, one's social mask. This is the structure that allows the child to interface with, and yet be protected from, the social world. A flexible persona allows the child to interact effectively with others in his or her world, while retaining his or her unique identity. An overly rigid persona, though, implies that the ego has become meshed with the persona, and the child *becomes* the mask of the "good girl" or the "tough guy," with no access to his or her inner uniqueness. On the other hand, some children fail to develop a persona at all, and remain completely unsocialized, developing no effective ways to defend themselves from their unconscious impulses, or any social skills to allow them to adapt to social norms and get their needs met in socially acceptable ways.

Another archetype that is important to recognize is the *Shadow*, which contains all that is not acceptable to the developing ego and persona, as well as those aspects of the conscious personality that have remained undeveloped, perhaps because they were not valued by the child's environment. The shadow splits itself off from consciousness and expresses itself in behavior that is disturbing and often destructive. However, the shadow is not entirely negative: it also contains the creative impulses of the psyche that, when activated, can greatly enrich the personality of the individual.

All Jungian therapists must have experienced their own in-depth analysis, as they primarily work out of the transference–countertransference paradigm, and are keenly attuned to and skillfully use these phenomena in their work with clients. Indeed, practitioners of all three theoretical models described here are required to have intensive training in their respective theories to be maximally helpful to their clients.

Most Jungians use a traditional fully equipped playroom, although some use separate containers to store special toys used by a particular child in the working out of his or her issues. Jungian therapists value the playroom and the relationship between themselves and the child as a container, a "temenos," a "free and protected space" (Kalff, 1980), where the child can play freely and safely, more or less as he or she wishes. Limits are set as necessary, and are tailored to the individual needs of each child. The Jungian belief is that the child will intuitively go to the areas of play that are integral to the expression of his or her struggles and development, and limits are set that allow maximum expression while protecting the container of the relationship. The therapist follows the lead of the child by reflecting or interpreting the meaning of the child's feelings, behaviors, and struggles. The therapist engages in role play assigned by the child, asking many questions to clarify the role the child wants the therapist to play, all the while maintaining an analytical attitude toward the meaning of the play to the child. Jungians believe that during the three phases of treatment, the child generally will progress through patterns in his or her play of chaos, struggle, and then resolution. In the temenos of the playroom, the child experiences a sanctuary from the demands of the external world where regression and then progression can occur. Here the child can begin to understand, accept, and transform painful affect into a healthier, more positive sense of self. The role of the therapist is to witness the child's unconscious process as it unfolds in play and through art expression, holding firm to the belief that the child will go to his or her problem areas, struggle with the "good versus bad" feelings, and slowly begin to develop mastery of these painful affects and a sense of inner control (Allan & Levin, 1993, pp. 211–212). The more directive element of Jungian play therapy involves encouraging the child to express his or her issues symbolically through various art and sandplay media, through movement and dance, and through journaling and other writings. This encouragement is used throughout all phases of Jungian play therapy.

STANDARD PLAY THERAPY ASSESSMENTS AND EVALUATION PROCEDURES

To our knowledge, there are no commonly used standard procedures for evaluating progress in play therapy. There are many instruments used to evaluate play, in terms of development, and diagnosis of children's play either individually, in groups, or in families (Gitlin-Weiner, Sandgrund, & Schaefer, 2000). O'Connor also uses, in his three phases of assessment for determining which objectives to use for each individual child seen in ecosystemic play therapy, an instrument called the Developmental Therapy Teaching Objectives Rating Form—Revised (DTORF-R, 4th ed.; O'Connor, 1997).

Three instruments mentioned in the literature have been developed to assess play behaviors of children in play therapy, although they have not been widely disseminated. The first is called the Play Behaviors Adjustment Rating Scale (PBARS), developed by Oe (1989). Oe looked at 10 types of play behaviors seen in play therapy (exploratory, incidental, creative or coping, dramatic or role, relationship building, relationship testing, self-accepting, self-rejecting, acceptance of environment, and nonacceptance of environment) and rated them in terms of frequency and intensity. She also investigated children's attitudes in play over three dimensions (positive, ambivalent, and negative), again as to frequency and intensity. This rating scale is completed upon observation of the videotape of a child's first play therapy session to determine areas of strength and weakness.

A second instrument is the Play Therapy Observational Instrument (PTOI), developed by Howe and Silvern (1981) and adapted by Perry (Perry & Landreth, 1991). It was designed to help in the assessment of a child's functioning in his or her environment, and to aid in treatment planning and rating of prognosis. Three areas of functioning were addressed (social inadequacy, emotional discomfort, and use of fantasy) in a 13-item questionnaire scored from 12-second segments of a videotaped play therapy session. It has shown promise in tracking changes in children's play during the treatment process (Gitlin-Weiner et al., 2000).

The third instrument, called the NOVA Assessment of Psychotherapy (NAP), was also designed to evaluate play therapy process and outcome (Faust & Burns, 1991). Seventeen child behaviors and 12 therapist behaviors are coded in 7-second intervals during a session of play therapy, involving four categories of behaviors (positive or negative affect expressed, cooperative behaviors, and aggressive behaviors). This instrument, too, may be useful for evaluating affective and behavioral changes during the therapy process (Gitlin-Weiner et al., 2000). None of these instruments has been involved in either normative or validation studies since their development, nor widely used in play therapy assessment or evaluation. However, each has promise in evaluating children's play therapy behaviors both for research and for diagnostic and prognostic purposes.

Family Play Assessment (FPA; Fagot & Kavanagh, 1991) assists the play therapist in understanding family dynamics and parental role-taking abilities. The FPA can be used at various times throughout the treatment process. It can be used as a needs assessment prior to parenting instruction, to identify the effectiveness of play therapy or parent training, to compare parenting styles and parent–child relationships in child custody cases, to assess for risk of physical abuse, and as a pre- and postmeasure for research. Additionally, it is useful to reduce resistance to counseling for both children and parents. As part of the intake process, the FPA provides insight into family dynamics at a depth not available during an interview.

The FPA is simple to set up and complete. It can take place in a clinic setting or in the family home. Research by Fagot and Kavanagh (1991) has indicated that the parents' behavior and interaction with their own child will be the same in either setting. During a structured 15–20 minute play session, the interaction between the parents and their children can be analyzed for the content of the play and to identify the affect and nature of interaction.

The play session has three distinct parts: (1) a decision process in which a shared activity is chosen, providing insight into the family's decision-making process; (2) 10 minutes of shared activity, providing an opportunity to observe interactions and the content of play; (3) a clean-up phase, providing insight into child compliance with parental requests. The play therapist instructs the parents:

> "I would like you and your children to *play together*. Try to relax and act normally. Please do *something together*. I'll let you know when you have 10 minutes left. At that time, I would like *you* to ask the children to put all the toys away. Okay, start."

Continue observing until all the toys are put away. If in a clinical setting, observe behind a two-way mirror or via videotape. If in the family home, sit separate from the family, such as in the doorway or a hallway.

Research by Fagot and Kavanagh (1991) identified critical incidents by which families at high risk for physical abuse could be identified. These include negative verbal behaviors directed toward the child, such as name calling; competing for resources, in which the parent acts like a sibling to her or his child with behaviors such as taking away toys; few positive interaction skills, such that parents feel the need to be in control of the child, but have few positive, and many negative, coercive behaviors in their repertoire; and low tolerance, where parents are obviously uncomfortable with the give-and-take that takes place in most families. The critical incident behaviors were not seen in 250 nonabusive families that participated in the Fagot and Kavanagh research.

CLINICAL APPLICATIONS
WITH CHILDREN AND FAMILIES

Just before 3-year-old Carrie leaned over to kiss my cheek and say "good night" she snuggled a large T-Rex dinosaur toy next to me. Following her previous directions, I was laying on the baby blanket Carrie had arranged on the playroom floor. She covered me with a second baby blanket and instructed me to "go to sleep." She turned on a "nightlight" (a toy camping lantern) to "keep me safe" and left me to "sleep" while she went to the playroom kitchen to "cook dinner for daddy." However, while this apparently tranquil home scene was happening (T-Rex aside!), Carrie instructed me to repeatedly say, "I'm scared" and to "cry."

Carrie and I were in the midst of a play therapy session. She was coming to play therapy because of night terrors she had experienced for more than a year, usually for five nights a week.

Carrie and I had a well-developed therapeutic relationship. She was used to being in charge, directing the play, taking the session where she needed it to go. I followed her lead and instructions. Carrie reenacted her bedtime, but in her play I was her and she was the parent. Carrie was trying to make sense of her nighttime experience. She was able to play the mommy who went about putting the child lovingly and safely to bed. She was able to experience being the person who was in charge, the caretaker, who competently carried on the family routine.

Carrie instructed me to be her, the child who was scared and crying, who snuggled down with a T-Rex dinosaur! Was the T-Rex a symbol of how afraid she felt, as if she slept with such overwhelming danger? Or was it a symbol of how much protection she needed? Was something out there so scary she needed a strong, ferocious T-Rex to keep her safe? Being nondirective I did not ask. I sensed what it was like to be in her world: I was her! What was I sensing, feeling, thinking, being in her world? My sense at that moment was that I was in danger. The T-Rex represented that danger. How could I be safe, even with a nightlight? I HAD A DINOSAUR IN BED WITH ME! No wonder I (Carrie) cried and was scared. But "Mommy" did not understand: She went off to fix dinner, leaving me alone with my danger.

Carrie and I played out this scenario for several weeks and the play changed. First, the T-Rex no longer went to bed with me. Next, she no longer instructed me to say I was scared or to cry. With these changes I began sensing changes in her world, so I began saying "I feel so safe mommy" and "I'm gonna sleep all night, no scary dreams tonight." She did not correct me. Carrie's mother soon reported that Carrie was sleeping well through the night. Carrie, with this issue resolved, began working on other issues during her play therapy sessions.

Charlie, 3½ years old, and Tiffany, 6 years old, had been participating in sibling play therapy. The sibling relationship had become difficult and at times combative. A major source of contention between Charlie and Tiffany was sharing their parents. When Charlie was born, the parents decided that the mother would be Charlie's primary caretaker and the father would become Tiffany's primary caretaker. Thus began the unusual subsystems within this family: father–daughter and mother–son.

When Charlie reached 2 years of age the parents decided to realign the parent–child subsystems: father–mother and daughter–son. Tiffany and Charlie were not excited about the change, to say the least.

During parent consultations the parents began reporting that sibling issues were greatly improved. However, the sibling issues were still very apparent in the sibling play therapy sessions. I was not convinced that the family functioning had improved as much as the parents reported. Consequently, I asked the family to participate in a family play session to assess overall interactions. They readily agreed.

The typical instructions were given for a family play assessment. The family was to play together for 15 minutes and the parents asked the children to clean up at the end of the session. What I observed through the two-way mirror confirmed my clinical hunches. Although asked to play together, the father went to the sandbox and the mother began painting at the easel. Both children attempted on several occasions to engage their parents in play. The parents, however, were focused on their own activities. After several attempts to engage their parents, Tiffany and Charlie began playing together. It appeared that there was real improvement in the child subsystem. However, the parents gave only token acknowledgment of their children's presence. As a result of this family play session I was able to make major changes in how I worked with them during parent consultations.

CONCLUSION

Play therapy has a rich history and diverse application. It provides children access to mental health services that take into account childhood developmental issues. As a result children are able to deal with disruptive life experiences and move forward in their lives. As play therapists, we are given the honor to walk through that therapeutic experience with them. Jointly we enter the child's world, communicate through the language of play, and together, play therapist and child client, we are forever changed.

REFERENCES

Allan, J. (1988). *Inscapes of the child's world.* Dallas, TX: Spring.

Allan, J. (1997). Jungian play psychotherapy. In K. J. O'Connor & L. M. Braverman (Eds.), *Play therapy theory and practice: A comparative presentation* (pp. 100–130). New York: Wiley.

Allan, J., & Berry, P. (1987). Sandplay. *Elementary School Guidance and Counseling, 21*(4), 300–306.

Allan, J., & Bertoia, J. (1992). *Written paths to healing: Education and Jungian child counseling.* Dallas, TX: Spring.

Allan, J., & Brown, K. (1993). Jungian play therapy in elementary schools. *Elementary School Guidance and Counseling, 28*(1), 30–41.

Allan, J., & Levin, S. (1993). 'Born on my bum': Jungian play therapy. In T. Kottman & C. Schaefer (Eds.), *Play therapy in action: A casebook for practitioners* (pp. 209–244). Northvale, NJ: Aronson.

Axline, V. (1947). *Play therapy: The inner dynamics of childhood.* Boston: Houghton Mifflin.

Axline, V. (1969). *Play therapy.* New York: Ballantine Books.

Axline, V. (1971). *Dibs: In search of self.* New York: Ballantine Books.

Bertoia, J. (1999). The invisible village: Jungian group play therapy. In D. Sweeney & L. Homeyer (Eds.), *The handbook of group play therapy* (pp. 86–104). San Francisco: Jossey-Bass.

Brody, V. (1993). *The dialogue of touch: Developmental play therapy.* Treasure Island, FL: Play Training Associates.

Carey, L. (1999). *Sandplay therapy with children and families.* Northvale, NJ: Aronson.

DeDomenico, G. (1994). Jungian play therapy techniques. In K. J. O'Connor & C. E. Schaefer (Eds.), *Handbook of play therapy: Volume 2. Advances and innovation* (pp. 253–282). New York: Wiley.

Fagot, B. I., & Kavanaugh, K. (1991). Play as a diagnostic tool with physically abusive parents and their children. In C. Schaefer, K. Gitlin, & A. Sandgrund (Eds.), *Play diagnosis and assessment* (pp. 203–218). New York: Wiley.

Faust, J., & Burns, W. (1991). Coding therapist and child interaction: Progress and outcome in play therapy. In C. Schaefer, K. Gitlin, & A. Sandgrund (Eds.), *Play diagnosis and assessment* (pp. 663–690). New York: Wiley.

Freud, A. (1965). *The psycho-analytic treatment of children.* New York: International Universities Press.

Ginott, H. (1961). *Group psychotherapy with children: The theory and practice of play therapy.* New York: McGraw-Hill.

Gitlin-Weiner, K., Sandgrund, A., & Schaefer, C. (Eds.). (2000). *Play diagnosis and assessment* (2nd ed.). New York: Wiley.

Guerney, L. (1969). *Psychotherapeutic agents: New roles for non-professionals, parents and teachers.* New York: Holt, Rinehart, & Winston.

Guerney, L. (1983). Introduction to filial therapy: Training parents as therapists. In P. Keller & L. Ritt (Eds.), *Innovations in clinical practice: A source book* (pp. 26–39). Sarasota, FL: Professional Resource Exchange.

Guerney, L. (1992). *Parenting: A skills training manual* (4th ed.). State College, PA: Ideals.

Guerney, L. (1993). Client-centered (nondirective) play therapy. In T. Kottman & C. Schaefer (Eds.), *Play therapy in action: A casebook for practitioners* (pp. 21–64). Northvale, NJ: Aronson.

Hambidge, G. (1955). Structured play therapy. *American Journal of Orthopsychiatry, 25,* 601–607.

Homeyer, L., & Sweeney, D. (1998). *Sandtray: A practical manual.* Canyon Lake, TX: Lindan Press.

Howe, P., & Silvern, L. (1981). Behavioral observation during play therapy: Preliminary development of a research instrument. *Journal of Personality Assessment, 45,* 168–182.

Hug-Hellmuth, H. (1921). On the technique of child-analysis. *International Journal of Psychoanalysis, 2,* 281–305.

Hunter, L. (1998). *Images of resiliency: Troubled children create healing stories in the language of the sandplay.* Palm Beach, FL: Behavioral Communications Institute.

Jernberg, A. (1979). *Theraplay: A new treatment using structured play for problem children and their families.* San Francisco: Jossey-Bass.

Kaduson, H., Cangelosi, D., & Schaefer, C. (1997). *The play cure: Individualized play therapy for specific childhood problems.* Northvale, NJ: Aronson.

Kalff, D. (1971). *Sandplay: Mirror of a child's psyche.* San Francisco: Browser Press.

Kalff, D. (1980). *Sandplay: A psychotherapeutic approach to the psyche.* Boston: Sigo Press.

Klein, M. (1932). *The psycho-analysis of children.* London: Hogarth Press.

Knell, S. (1993). *Cognitive-behavioral play therapy.* Northvale, NJ: Aronson.

Kottman, T. (1987). An ethnographic study of an Adlerian play therapy training program. *Dissertation Abstracts International, A49*(01).

Kottman, T. (1993). The king of rock and roll: An application of Adlerian play therapy. In T. Kottman & C. Schaefer (Eds.), *Play therapy in action: A casebook for practitioners* (pp. 133–168). Northvale, NJ: Aronson.

Kottman, T. (1994). Adlerian play therapy. In K. J. O'Connor & C. E. Schaefer (Eds.), *Handbook of play therapy: Vol. 2. Advances and innovations* (pp. 3–26). New York: Wiley.

Kottman, T. (1995). *Partners in play: An Adlerian approach to play therapy.* Alexandria, VA: American Counseling Association.

Kottman, T. (1997). Adlerian play therapy. In K. J. O'Connor & L. M. Braverman (Eds.), *Play therapy theory and practice: A comparative presentation* (pp. 310–340). New York: Wiley.

Kottman, T. (1999). Integrating the crucial C's into Adlerian play therapy. *Journal of Individual Psychology, 55*(3), 288–297.

Kottman, T. (2001). *Play therapy: Basics and beyond.* Alexandria, VA: American Counseling Association.

Kottman, T., & Johnson, V. (1993). Adlerian play therapy: A tool for school counselors. *Elementary School Guidance and Counseling, 28*(1), 42–51.

Kottman, T., & Stiles, K. (1990). The mutual storytelling technique: An Adlerian application in child therapy. *Journal of Individual Psychology, 46*(2), 148–156.

Kottman, T., & Warlick, J. (1989). Adlerian play therapy: Practical considerations. *Journal of Individual Psychology, 45*(4), 433–446.

Kottman, T., & Warlick, J. (1990). Adlerian play therapy. *Journal of Humanistic Education and Development, 28*, 125–132.

Landreth, G. (1991). *Play therapy: Art of the relationship.* Muncie, IN: Accelerated Development.

Landreth, G., & Sweeney, D. (1997). Child-centered play therapy. In K. O'Connor & L. M. Braverman (Eds.), *Play therapy theory and practice: A comparative presentation* (pp. 17–45). New York: Wiley.

Levy, D. (1933). Use of the play technique as experimental procedure. *American Journal of Orthopsychiatry, 3*, 266–277.

Levy, D. (1939). "Release therapy" in young children. *Psychiatry, 1*, 387–390.

Lilly, J. P. (2003, October). *Jungian play therapy.* Paper presented at the meeting of the Association for Play Therapy, Kansas City, KA.

Lowenfeld, M. (1993). *Understanding children's sandplay: Lowenfeld's World Technique.* Aylesbury, UK: Margaret Lowenfeld Trust.

Moustakas, C. (1953). *Children in play therapy: A key to understanding normal and disturbed emotions.* New York: McGraw-Hill.

Moustakas, C. (1966). *Existential child therapy: The child's discovery of himself.* New York: Basic Books.

Moustakas, C. (1992). *Psychotherapy with children: The living relationships.* Greeley, CO: Carron.

Norton, C. C., & Norton, B. E. (1997). *Reaching children through play therapy: An experiential approach.* Denver, CO: Publishing Cooperative.

Oaklander, V. (1988). *Windows to our children: A Gestalt therapy approach to our children and adolescents.* New York: Gestalt Journal.

O'Connor, K. (1991). *The play therapy primer: An integration of theories and techniques.* New York: Wiley.

O'Connor, K. (1997). Ecosystemic play therapy. In K. O'Connor & C. Schaefer (Eds.), *Play therapy primer* (pp. 234–284). New York: Wiley.

O'Connor, K. (2000). *The play therapy primer* (2nd ed.). New York: Wiley.

O'Connor, K., & Ammen, S. (1997). *Play therapy treatment planning and interventions: The ecosystemic model and workbook.* San Diego: CA: Academic Press.

Oe, E. (1989). Comparison of initial session play therapy behaviors of maladjusted and adjusted children. *Dissertation Abstracts International, A50*(09).

Perry, L. (1993). Audrey, the bois d'arc and me: A time of becoming. In T. Kottman & C. Schaefer (Eds.), *Play therapy in action: A casebook for practitioners* (pp. 5–44). Northvale, NJ: Aronson.

Perry, L., & Landreth, G. (1991). Diagnostic assessment of children's play therapy behavior. In C. Schaefer, K. Gitlin, & A. Sandgrund (Eds.), *Play diagnosis and assessment* (pp. 631–660). New York: Wiley.

Rogers, C. (1951). *Client-centered therapy.* Boston: Houghton Mifflin.

Solomon, J. (1938). Active play therapy. *American Journal of Orthopsychiatry, 8*(3), 763–781.

Sweeney, D., & Homeyer, L. (1999). *The handbook of group play therapy.* San Francisco: Jossey-Bass.

VanFleet, R. (1994). *Filial therapy: Strengthening parent–child relationships through play.* Sarasota, FL: Professional Resource Press.

Wells, H. G. (1911). *Floor games.* New York: Arno Press.

≈ 8

Sandtray Therapy

LINDA E. HOMEYER
DANIEL S. SWEENEY

The tools of the sandtray therapist are simple: *sand and water*, which are basic elements of the earth; a *tray*, in which to contain the work; and a *collection of miniatures*, which serve as a universe of symbols and images. These simple tools are, however, only elements of the process. Using these effectively with clients—that is the *craft* of the sandtray therapist.

Homeyer and Sweeney (1998) define *sandtray therapy* as "an expressive and projective mode of psychotherapy involving the unfolding and processing of intra- and inter-personal issues through the use of specific sandtray materials as a nonverbal medium of communication, led by the client(s) and facilitated by a trained therapist" (p. 6). The therapeutic use of sand in a tray, with a collection of miniatures and the availability of water, has been used in a variety of ways since its inception.

BRIEF HISTORY

Margaret Lowenfeld (1979) sought a method to connect with children in an honest way, without contaminating the child's communication with adult perceptions, perspectives, or preconceived theories. As a medical doctor in the Russo–Polish War (1920), Lowenfeld was profoundly influenced by the horrors and impact of war on the troops, prisoners of war, displaced students, children, and families she witnessed and treated. When Lowenfeld began working with children in 1925, she sought to develop a method through which children could communicate their perception of their world. Lowenfeld sought "to find a medium which would in itself be instantly attractive to children and which would give them and the observer a 'language,' as it were, through which communication could be easily established" (1979, p. 281). She recalled reading a book, *Floor Games*, by H. G. Wells (1911). In the book Wells shares the lengthy and involved stories he and his sons would play with small toys on the floor of his home. So, with an initial collection of small toys, Lowenfeld offered children a chance to share their worlds with her. Her system became known as the "World Technique."

The next and second major force in the use of sandtray was Dora Kalff. Kalff, after attending the Jung Institute for 6 years, attended a psychiatric conference where she heard Lowenfeld present her World Technique (Weinrib, 1983). In 1935, Kalff went to London and studied with Lowenfeld. She returned to Switzerland and developed the technique she called "Sandplay" (Kalff, 1980). Kalff was influenced by Jung's mentoring and her experience with Eastern mysticism while living in the Far East.

It is important to note that the term *sandplay* is frequently misused to describe *any* psychotherapeutic use of the sandtray and miniatures. The term *sandplay*, however, specifically applies to the Jungian approach to sandtray therapy. While the approaches of Lowenfeld and Kalff remain the primary approaches to the therapeutic use of the sandtray (to be further discussed below), other orientations have been developed over the past several decades.

Oaklander (1988) employs a Gestalt approach to working with clients in the sandtray. She posits that sand and play therapy interventions assist in the formulation of an I/Thou relationship, a key concept in Gestalt therapy (Oaklander, 1994). Further, as a process therapy, Gestalt sandtray therapy enables clients to process contact-boundary disturbances and to create a sense of self that may have been damaged, promote awareness, and address resistance (Oaklander, 1994).

DeDomenico (1995, 1999) developed the method called "Sandtray-Worldplay." Her initial research was with normal preschool children in nondirective sandtray. The children worked in individual trays in a group setting. She discovered the preschoolers could work 2–4 hours, creating a series of evolving worlds. She now works extensively with sandtray in individual and group settings, with clients working in parallel, joint, and communal play. A proponent of group sandtray, DeDomenico (1999) indicates that group provides clients with the opportunity to develop the "ability and interest to create communally" (p. 220), and that the group sandtray experience can "overshadow the individual's separate identity. . . . Sandtray becomes a true mirror of the group psyche and what community is really about" (p. 220).

MAJOR THEORETICAL ORIENTATIONS

As noted, the two primary approaches to sandtray therapy work are based on the work of Lowenfeld and Kalff. These are briefly described and compared in this section; a more detailed discussion of the eclectic approach used by the authors follows later in the chapter. The interested reader is referred to *The World Technique* (Lowenfeld, 1979) and *Sandplay* (Kalff, 1980) for further description and explanation.

Lowenfeld (1979) was interested in exploring the processes of the child's mind when she developed the World Technique. The internal world of the child's experience was the focus of her work. Although trained first as a pediatrician and later psychoanalytically, Lowenfeld did not try to fit the child's creation in the sandtray into existing theoretical constructs. Indeed, in some ways, she made the first attempt at being child-centered. Lowenfeld did not direct a child's selection of miniatures or creation of the tray. Lowenfeld viewed the tray as both a communication from the child to the therapist and a communication to the child's self.

Kalff (1980) focused on what she termed the "free and protected space" for the child and the creation in the sand. She felt that the client needed to be free to express anything and everything, and that the media and the therapist needed to provide a protected space with which and with whom the child felt safe to express his or her self. The therapist was responsible for creating this space, and together with the media served as the psychological and physical "container" for the client.

While there are many similarities between the World Technique and Sandplay, there are some fundamental differences that are helpful to consider. The following are summarized from Lowenfeld (1979) and Kalff (1980), and are certainly open to interpretation. It should be noted that many therapists who practice sandtray therapy do not adhere strictly to either perspective. Consider the following comparisons:

- In both the World Technique and Sandplay, the goal is to uncover nonverbal material. In Sandplay the focus is on the totality of the unconscious psyche, whereas in the World Technique the focus is on nonverbal consciousness.

- The therapeutic benefit of Sandplay involves the healing power of the client's psyche (including metaphorical symbols and archetypes), which is viewed (reverenced) by the therapist (guide). Considerable weight is given to the internal wisdom of the client. The World Technique gives greater involvement and power to the therapist, in that the dialogue about the tray focuses on insight and psychodynamic processes. It might be argued that Sandplay puts greater focus on the client's ego, while the World Technique focuses on the therapist lending ego strength to the client through the therapeutic relationship.

- Thus, there is greater involvement of the therapist in the World Technique. The Lowenfeld therapist will sit close to the traymaker and frequently talk or dialog with the client. The focus is on the creation and the creative process as a picture of the client's world, and the therapist is much more involved. Sandplay therapists would also observe, but do so less obviously, because they consider a more active role intrusive. The focus seems to be more on the finished product than on the creative process.

- In the discussion of the tray and its creation, Lowenfeld therapists make direct connections between the tray, the miniatures, and the client's life. There are questions, comments, and interpretations. Sandplay therapists listen to the client's story, but in an observer role. While Kalff herself cautioned against interpretation, many Sandplay therapists interpret symbols and archetypes quite frequently. Kalff would argue that the greater the verbal involvement of the therapist, the less likely that unconscious connections can be made.

- The World Technique included miniatures that were primarily stored in drawers. This might attest to Lowenfeld's greater focus on nonverbal conscious material, as the client would arguably require more conscious intent in the creation process. This is contrasted with the Sandplay approach of displaying miniatures on open shelves, so that the client can unconsciously be "caught" by metaphorical images. The World Technique also included a standardization of miniatures and process, as diagnosis and research were a greater focus. There is no standardization for Sandplay, and there also is not a diagnostic or research focus.

There are other comparisons that might be made between the work of Lowenfeld and Kalff. What is important to recognize is that both approaches are probably more similar than they are different. They both focus on allowing client issues to unfold nonverbally. As with other expressive therapies described in this book, the application of any sandtray approach can be a powerful healing experience.

ASSESSMENT AND EVALUATION WITH THE SANDTRAY

Sandtray is used primarily therapeutically, rather than diagnostically. Although clinicians initially studied sandtray as a projective and diagnostic technique, clinicians currently prefer the therapeutic application (Mitchell & Friedman, 1994). A brief overview of the diagnostic uses are covered below. This summary will provide the reader with a richer understanding of the development of sandtray. Additionally, insight into clinical implications of research are noted.

Developmental Research

Understanding how nonclinical, or "normal," individuals work in the sandtray is important to identifying features of the sandtray that have clinical implications. How does one know if a client is working at a regressed level without understanding age-appropriate work? Early developmental studies provide this information.

Charlotte Buhler's (1951a) research initially focused on establishing developmental norms for work done in sandtrays. Buhler's work was originally named the "World Test" and later the "Toy World Test" to more clearly differentiate her work from that of her colleague, Margaret Lowenfeld. Table 8.1 includes Buhler's developmental findings along with those of Bowyer (1970) and Jones (1983).

Clinical Assessments

Buhler's (1951a, 1951b) work also resulted in identifying signs, or symptoms, of client emotional disturbance in the sandtray. Lowenfeld's and Buhler's work, and that of others who followed, resulted in the development of "classic worlds" tray organization identified as the Empty World, the Unpeopled World, the Aggressive World, the Closed World, Worlds with Rows, and Disorganized Worlds. Buhler indicated that all subjects typically showed one sign; two or more of these signs

TABLE 8.1. Developmental Norm Studies

Age (years)	Developmental norms
2–3	• Uses front horizontal edge and the left corner of the tray in which to place figures (Bowyer, 1970). • Plays with toys on the floor and fetches toys from around the room; may fling or poke toys into the sand (Bowyer, 1980). • Inclined to pick up jungle animals first while expressing excitement (Bowyer, 1970). • Does not exhibit control as illustrated by chaotic World scenes (Bowyer, 1970); chaotic massing of figures (Jones, 1983). • Reveals an emerging sense of perspective (Jones, 1983). • Most figures are placed within the boundaries of the tray, but often some are also placed outside the tray (Jones, 1983). • Most of the tray is used but it is not uncommon for only part of the tray to be used (Jones, 1983). • Depending on the level of involvement in dramatic play, use and orientation of figures might be intentional or unintentional (Jones, 1983). • Boundaries may appear without apparent intentionality (Jones, 1983). • Sand is primarily used for burying and unburying figures (Jones, 1983).
4	• Typically poured sand over people or thing or pushed object into the sand (Bowyer, 1970). • Constructed scenes that showed an increase in coherent detail (Bowyer, 1970). • Four year olds included a number of traffic signs and sometimes included a police officer (Bowyer, 1970). • Children between the ages of 4 and 6 engaged in dramatic activity—e.g., making zooming noises with airplanes (Bowyer, 1970).
5	• Exhibited a preoccupation with having enough food for the people and farm animals (Bowyer, 1970). • Eating themes were prevalent (Bowyer, 1970). • Used people and animals proportionately (Bowyer, 1970). • Children older than 5 commonly constructed farm scenes and included numerous animals in their scene and utilized the whole tray (Bowyer, 1970).
7	• Typically played out a cowboy and Indian theme with opposing forces being apparent (Bowyer, 1970). • Utilized the sand to construct hills, valleys, roads, and tunnels. (This type of construction was rarely seen in younger children.) • Often constructed peaceful farm scenes. • Often included a number of trees. • The number of miniatures used increased concurrently with increasing age (Buhler, 1951a). • Girls indicated more symptoms than boys (Buhler, 1951a). • By age 8 (or earlier) construction is created with a basic plan that is then filled in with the details. Typically the initial layout includes houses, fences, or the bridge. • 91–100% of the tray is used (Jones, 1983).
8	• Figures used in three significant ways: manipulated in motion; used to create and play a game; used to construct scenes or buildings (Buhler, 1951a).

(*continued*)

TABLE 8.1. (*continued*)

Age (years)	Developmental norms
	• When more than two figures are used, dramatic grouping is simple (e.g., two witches around a caldron); dramatic action between figure is obvious in terms of placement, action, relationship between figures (Jones, 1983). • A partial construction is seen that reflects beginnings of various relationships; two figures are purposefully oriented and are interpersonally and functionally related (Jones, 1983). • Younger children frequently included fencing in their scene, typically created smaller worlds and constructed rows (Buhler, 1951a). • No children excluded cars or people in their play (Buhler, 1951a). • It is common to see two or more symptoms* in construction of children up to age 6 (Buhler, 1951a). • The world is created within the confines of the tray (Jones, 1983).
10	• Emphasis on factual and realistic scenes (Bowyer, 1970). • Children carefully chose the miniatures and rejected some because of their disproportionate size to their scene (Bowyer, 1970). • Fencing is frequently seen (Bowyer, 1970). • Coherent world typically vies with a single concrete theme (Jones, 1983). • Objects are grouped in meaningful relationships that include symmetry. • Figures are within confines of the tray (Jones, 1983). • Orientation of figures is intentional, and scale and placement become important (Jones, 1983). • Some dramatic play occurs, usually centered on the cooperation between figures (Jones, 1983). • Increased complexity of classification—for example, human neighborhood are clearly portrayed (Jones, 1983). • Boundaries are defined by figures that are somewhat clear, or no boundary figures are present (Jones, 1983). • 91–100% of the tray is used (Jones, 1983).
10–12	• Children older than 11 frequently included trees (Bowyer, 1970).
12–18	• Children typically constructed scenes of a town or village that included a school, church, or both, or a landscape along with a human settlement (Bowyer, 1970). • Figures displaying the human community are clearly established or an integrated, lone figure may be used (Jones, 1983). • Symbolic and realistic worlds are created and characterized by (a) a single theme encompassing a complex part that may not be completely integrated; (b) an abstract theme uniting seemingly unrelated figures; or (c) a single clear theme with parts exhibiting interdependence and integration (Jones, 1983). • Figures are within confines of the tray (Jones, 1983). • No dramatic play occurs (Jones, 1983). • 91–100% of the tray is used (Jones, 1983). • Boundaries are also created by well-coordinated groupings of miniatures, which may relate to a complex world (Jones, 1983). • Sand is extensively used to create land and water forms, as well as boundaries (Jones, 1983).

Note. Compiled by Petruk (1997). Adapted by permission of the author.
*Buhler's symptoms of emotional disturbance. See the list on p. 169.

within one tray indicated emotional disturbance. The six classifications of signs or symptoms and their possible clinical meanings are as follows:

I. Unpeopled Worlds: No people are in the sandtray. This is seen as especially true when the client puts in *only* soldiers.
   A. A disturbance in social relationships
   B. Projection of escape wishes
   C. Hostile feelings toward people
II. Empty Worlds: When one-third or more of the tray is not used or empty. May also be defined as less than 50 items/miniatures and use of less than five categories of miniatures.
   A. Cannot access mental resources because of depression or other deficiency
   B. Expression that the client's world is an unhappy, empty place
   C. Meagerness of ideas
   D. Desire for rejection and escape of things
III. Disorganized, Chaotic Worlds: Items placed without any order.
   A. Signs of impulsivity
   B. Reflects inner confusion, dissolution
   C. Breakdown of ego organization
IV. Rigid Worlds/Worlds with Rows: Particularly overexaggerated uniformity.
   A. Projection of either primitive or perfectionistic attempts to create order
   B. Obsessive need for self-control
   C. Emotional rigidity and repression
V. Fenced/Closed Worlds: Most of the construction is closed in.
   A. Self-protective, closing off from others
   B. Closing dangers out
   C. Fear of own inner impulses, need for external control
VI. Aggressive World: Use of aggressive items, soldiers, cannons, wild animal attacks, games where people got killed or died, car crashes.
   A. Projection of strong feelings of aggression

Lumry's (1951) research validated Buhler's earlier research. None of her population of normal subjects displayed more than one of the above signs or symptoms. As in Buhler's work, her clinical population showed two or more signs. Currently, rather than using the above signs or symptoms to diagnose or identify emotional disturbance, the signs are used to provide clinical insight for use within the therapeutic process.

Bowyer (1970) suggested the following degree or level of regression and implications for each of the above worlds: (1) Empty Worlds, 2–4 years, difficult to treat children as they tend to withdraw, exhibit apathy, or lack mental capacity; (2) Disorganized/Chaotic Worlds, 2–5 years, sometimes result from aggressive play, similar implications as Empty Worlds, but not as severe; (3) Fenced Worlds, 8 years and older, lack of gates indicates less maturity; (4) Rigid Worlds, 8 years or older, unless displayed by rows of unrealistic objects, indicating less maturity; (5) Unpeopled Worlds cannot be identified as any level of regression as no "normal" children of any age range excluded people. Bowyer also only called trays unpeopled if they had neither people nor animals, as children often use animals to depict people.

Erik Erikson (1951) developed the Dramatic Perceptions Test (DPT) while working at Harvard. (This research was published under the name of Erik Homberger, his name before he changed it to Erikson [Homberger, 1938]). Erikson believed that children's play is a visual and sensory expression of their lives that precedes the development of verbalization (Stevens, 1983). His original study was designed to explore human development and character formation. His subjects were Harvard students who depicted traumatic events from their childhood. Erikson believed the conflicts that appeared in the scenes indicated that the students had picked up with their play at the point they had left off as children. He viewed these constructions as the students' attempt to repetitively play out the trauma to resolve their early traumatic experiences (Homberger, 1938; Petruk, 1996).

Others researched variations of the sandtray technique as a diagnostic method. These include the Toy World Test by Hedda Bolgar and Liosletter Fischer, the Sceno Test by Gerdhild von Stabbas, the Miniature Toy Interview by Lois Barclay Murphy, the Village Test by Henri Arthus and Pierre Mabille, and the Test of Imaginary Village by Mucchielli (cited in Mitchell & Friedman, 1994). None of these methods of assessment, however, has stood the test of time.

The Erica Method by Gosta Harding is reported to be widely used in Sweden and Scandinavia (Harding, 1947; Sjolund, 1981, 1993). Based on Buehler's World Test, the Erica Method is a projective technique used for assessment of the child's inner world. The child attends three sessions during which his or her process of building the world and the content of the created scene is analyzed. The Erica Method uses a standardized sandtray, set of miniatures, score sheet, and instructions. Sjolund (1981) asserts that the Erica Method "will provide comprehensive and meaningful information as to both developmental levels and psychological and psycho-pathological process" (p. 324).

Harding (1947) provided three considerations regarding children's sandtray constructions. She reminds us that (1) the World may represent the child's real situation; (2) the World may represent something the child longs for or dreams of; or (3) the World may be a symbolic expression of what is going on inside the child and not relate to any external situation, existing or desired.

SANDTRAY THERAPY PRINCIPLES IN PRACTICE

Sandtray, like any other technique, should be used in a thoughtful, purposeful, and intentional manner within the ongoing therapeutic milieu. Sandtray may be used in individual therapy (with children, adolescents, or adults), couple counseling, family therapy, and group counseling. It can be used as the primary mode of counseling, as a change of pace, or as a way of noting change and therapeutic progress. A brief discussion of the rationale and process of sandtray use and two case examples follows.

Rationale

The primary reason to use sandtray therapy is to assist clients who need a nonverbal method of dealing with their issues. Homeyer and Sweeney (1998) detail multiple rationales for the use of sandtray therapy. These include:

1. *Sandtray therapy gives expression to nonverbalized emotional issues.* Since play is the language of childhood, as well as a language for a client of any age who is unable or unwilling to verbalize, the sandtray provides a safe medium for expression. If play is the language, then the miniatures are the words. Just as an empty canvas provides a place for the artist's creative expression, so the tray provides a place for the client's emotional expression. The client needs no creative or artistic ability since the medium provides a flow that is free from evaluation.

The self-directed sandtray process allows clients to be fully themselves. Through the process of sandtray therapy, which includes a caring and accepting relationship, children and families can express their total personality. This enables hurting clients to consider new possibilities, some of which are not possible through verbal expression, and thus significantly develop the expression of self. Sandtray therapy is therefore more than a symbolization of the psyche, it is a forum for full self-expression and self-exploration.

2. *Sandtray therapy has a unique kinesthetic quality.* Sandtray therapy provides this sensory experience, and meets the need that we all (not just our clients) have for kinesthetic experiences. This fundamental essential, an extension of very basic attachment needs, is met through relationship and experience. Sandtray therapy provides both of these elements for clients.

The very tactile experience of touching and manipulating the sand is a therapeutic experience in and of itself. We have frequently met with nonverbal clients who have done nothing more than run their fingers through the sand, and then begin to talk about deep issues. It is as if the sensory experience with the sand causes a loosening of the tongue. The manipulation of the sand and the placement of the miniatures is both safe and kinesthetically satisfying, especially for clients whose prior sensory experiences were noxious.

3. *Sandtray therapy serves to create a necessary therapeutic distance for clients.* The client or family in emotional crisis is often unable to express his, her, or their pain in words, but may find expression through a projective medium such as sandtray therapy. It is simply easier for a traumatized client to "speak" through one of the sandtray therapy miniatures than to directly verbalize his or her pain. The consistency of the medium, and the consistency of the therapist in allowing the client to direct the process, creates a place where the client establishes the degree of therapeutic distance. Children, adults, and families in sandtray therapy may experience emotional release through symbolization and sublimation, through the projection onto the tray and miniatures.

4. *This therapeutic distance that sandtray therapy provides creates a safe place for abreaction to occur.* Children and families who have experienced trauma need a therapeutic setting in which to abreact, a place where repressed issues can emerge and be relived, as well as to experience the negative emotions that are frequently attached. Abreaction, a crucial element in the treatment of trauma, finds facilitated expression.

Schaefer (1994) suggested several properties that provide the sense of distance and often reluctant safety that children and families gain in sandtray therapy: (a) *symbolization*—for example, clients can use a predatory miniature to represent an abuser; (b) *"as-if" quality*—clients can use the pretend quality of sandtray therapy to act out events as if they are not real life; (c) *projection*—clients can project intense emotions onto the miniatures, who can then safely act out these feelings; and (d) *displacement*—clients can displace negative feelings onto the miniatures rather than expressing them toward family members. Sandtray therapy not only provides the opportunity for abreaction to occur, but facilitates the process through the setting and the media.

5. *Sandtray therapy with families is a truly inclusive experience.* An adult "talk" therapy approach to treating families is decidedly exclusive because it fails to recognize and honor the developmental level of children in the family. Sandtray therapy with families overcomes this obstacle. Sandtray therapy creates a "level playing field" for every family member, giving each person the opportunity to express him- or herself.

6. *Sandtray therapy naturally provides boundaries and limits, which promote safety for the client.* Boundaries and limits define the therapeutic relationship, as well as any other relationship. The careful structure of the sandtray therapy process and the carefully selected tools of the sandtray therapist provide the client with the boundaries that create the sense of safety he or she needs for growth. The size of the sandtray, the size and selection of miniatures, the office setting, and the guidance/instruction of the therapist all provide boundaries and limits for the client. While these limits are imperative and intentional, they promote freedom for expression. These inherent limits to sandtray therapy bring a focus to the therapeutic process, which in addition to promoting the safety that boundaries bring, assists the client in focusing on the therapeutic issues that need to be addressed.

7. *Sandtray therapy provides a unique setting for the emergence of therapeutic metaphors.* There is an increasing amount of literature on metaphors and psychotherapy, much of which focuses on verbal metaphors. Siegelman (1990) suggests that metaphors "combine the abstract and the concrete in a special way, enabling us to go from the known and the sensed to the unknown, and the symbolic. . . . They achieve this combination in a way that typically arises from and produces strong feeling that leads to integrating insight" (p. ix). Indeed, metaphors can be therapeutically powerful. We would suggest that the most powerful metaphors in therapy are those that are generated by the clients themselves. Sandtray therapy creates a consummate setting for this to occur. The sand and miniatures are ideal for clients to express their own therapeutic metaphors.

When therapeutic metaphors emerge, there naturally follows a therapeutic interpretation. We would echo Kalff's (1980) warning against focusing on interpretation, recognizing that it is the client's own interpretation that is the most important. We would further suggest that interpretation of sandtrays is not essential to the healing process. We often need to remind ourselves that when we interpret, we do so with our own minds and experiences, not with those of client. It is a helpful reminder that when interpreting a client's expression of an experience that the sharing of the interpretation is meant to serve the client's need and not the therapist's need.

8. *Sandtray therapy is effective in overcoming client resistance.* Sandtray therapy, because of its nonthreatening and engaging qualities, can captivate the involuntary client and draw in the reticent family member. Since play is the natural medium of communication for children, the child client who has been compelled into therapy by an adult is generally amenable to treatment because he or she is being allowed to express his or her self through play.

For the resistant individual or family member, sandtray therapy provides a means of communicating that diverts the fear of verbal conflict. The level of contribution that each family member makes to the construction of the sandtray may be a reflection of his or her investment in the family. In this regard, resistance not only can be overcome by sandtray therapy, but more fully identified as well.

9. *Sandtray therapy provides a needed and effective communication medium for the client with poor verbal skills.* Providing young children with a nonverbal therapeutic medium is a developmental necessity. Moreover, there are clients of all ages who have poor verbal skills, for a variety of reasons. Those with poor verbal skills include clients who experience developmental language delays or deficits, clients with social or relational difficulties, clients with physiological challenges, and others.

Just as the toddler who wants something desperately but cannot communicate this want to the parent, so can anyone have a great level of frustration when unable to effectively communicate needs. When the toddler has a tantrum because he cannot communicate his want or need to his parent, there is a vivid relationship challenge between child and parent. In the same way, relationship challenges of many types emerge in families when people are not able to verbalize their wants and needs. The sandtray therapy process creates a place where expression of needs and wants is not dependent upon words. The client with poor verbal skills, regardless of its etiology, finds a place of relief in sandtray therapy—a place where expression does not depend upon verbal acuity, but arises naturally through the freedom of the medium.

10. *Conversely, sandtray therapy cuts through verbalization used as a defense.* For the pseudomature child who presents as verbally astute yet is developmentally unable to effectively communicate on a cognitive level, sandtray therapy provides a means to communicate through the child's true and natural medium of communication. For the verbally sophisticated adult, who uses intellectualization and rationalization as a defense, sandtray therapy may cut through these defenses. This is an important dynamic to be aware of, since a family system that includes a verbally well-defended member also includes one or more members unable to establish effective communication and relationship. The nonverbal and expressive nature of sandtray therapy identifies this dynamic and provides a nonverbal way to address it.

11. *Sandtray therapy creates a place for the child client or family to experience control.* One of the primary results of crisis and trauma is a loss of control for people in its midst. The loss of emotional, psychological, and even physiological control is one of the most distressing byproducts of crisis and conflict. Both the individual and the family in crisis feel the frustration and fear of having lost control. A crucial goal for these clients must be to empower them, following any personal or family trauma that has been disempowering.

The self-directed process of sandtray therapy creates a place for control to be returned to the client. For the client looking to attain and extend self-control, sandtray therapy establishes the boundaries and allows the freedom for this to occur. For the client attempting to avoid responsibility, the sandtray therapy process places the responsibility for and control of the process on the client. If one goal of therapy is to help clients achieve a greater internal locus of control, sandtray therapy is an effective means toward this end.

12. *The challenge of transference may be effectively addressed through sandtray therapy.* The presence of an expressive medium creates an alternative object of transference. Lowenfeld (1979) proposed that through the creation of worlds in the sand, transference occurred between the client and the tray, rather than between the client and the therapist. Weinrib (1983) noted that the sandtray often becomes an independent object, so that the client may take away images of the tray rather than images of the therapist. Regardless of one's theoretical view of transference, however, sandtray therapy provides a means for transference issues to be safely addressed as needed. The tray and miniatures

may become objects of transference, or they may become the means by which transference issues are safely addressed.

13. *Deeper intrapsychic issues may be accessed more thoroughly and more rapidly through sandtray therapy.* Access to underlying emotional issues and unconscious conflicts is a challenge for any counselor. Although certainly not a comprehensive list, the qualities of sandtray therapy that have been suggested above generate an atmosphere where deep and complex intrapsychic issues can be safely approached.

Most clients have some level of motivation to change, as reflected by their presence in psychotherapy. Most of these clients likewise are often well defended when confronting challenges to their ego, which has already been injured. Sandtray therapy serves to decrease ego controls and other defenses and foster greater levels of disclosure. This in turn creates an increased capacity to consider interpersonal and intrapersonal alternatives.

Process

In Homeyer and Sweeney (1998) we discuss an eclectic approach to sandtray therapy. In the following section we offer a brief summary of our system. It begins with a discussion of the necessary equipment.

The media used in sandtray therapy may be very rudimentary or quite elaborate and detailed. It should not be considered essential to invest a great deal of office space or thousands of dollars in building an adequate collection of sandtray miniatures, as many therapists have done. The basic materials needed include two sandtrays and a selection of miniatures.

The sandtrays themselves are usually 20″ × 30″ × 3″, painted blue on the inside to simulate sky and water, and are half filled with fine sand. It is best not to use playground sand, which often contains small pebbles, or sand that is too fine, as it ends up being like powder. The size of the tray is important, primarily to provide boundaries and limits for the client and so that the contents of the tray can be viewed in a single glance. Two trays are desirable, and should be waterproof, so that one can be used for wet sand and the other for dry sand. The tray(s) should be set on a stable surface, preferably a table about average desk height, with room around the base of the tray. It may help to store tray(s) on a mobile cart that can be moved from the corner of the therapy room to the middle so clients can work with it.

A selection of miniatures is made available for use in the sand. It is generally suggested that miniatures be 2–3 inches in height. They should be selected exclusively for the sandtray therapy process—not collected. Again, thousands of miniatures are not necessary, but it is helpful to offer a wide assortment of toys and objects. Some basic categories include the following:

- Buildings (e.g., houses, castles, factories, schools, churches, stores)
- People (e.g., various racial/ethnic groups, soldiers, cowboys, sports figures, fantasy and mythological figures, various occupations)
- Vehicles (e.g., cars, trucks, planes, boats, emergency vehicles, farm equipment, military vehicles)
- Animals (e.g., domestic, farm, zoo, wild, marine, prehistoric)
- Vegetation (e.g., trees, shrubs, plants)
- Religious symbols (e.g., cross, madonna, menorah, nativity scene)
- Structures (e.g., fences, bridges, gates, highway signs)
- Natural objects (e.g., rocks, shells, driftwood, feathers)
- Miscellaneous (e.g., jewelry, wishing well, treasure chest)

Sensitivity to issues of diversity should be a priority in the selection of miniatures. Primarily, it is important to have miniature people of both genders who reflect a variety of ethnocultural groups. Using sandtray therapy in a predominately Asian community with a miniature collection containing only Caucasian figures would be totally inappropriate. Another sensitivity issue is geographical consistency; it is better to have miniature cactuses when working in a desert community and pine trees when working in a forest town.

Miniatures should be grouped together by category, and preferably displayed upon open shelves. Clients are less likely to rummage through drawers or bins than they are to select objects from a shelf. Consideration should also be given to categorization of the miniatures—for example, an emotionally fragile client is less likely to select a kitten set right next to a fire-breathing dragon. Furthermore, the impatient and reticent client may be unwilling to search through a disorganized shelf. A multiuse counseling office might necessitate a covered bookcase to hold miniatures, so they will not be a distraction to clients when not in use.

Homeyer and Sweeney (1998) describe six phases of the sandtray therapy process, including (1) preparation of the sandtray setting; (2) introduction of the process to the client; (3) creation of the sandtray; (4)

postcreation phase; (5) sandtray cleanup; and (6) documentation of the session.

Preparation of the sandtray setting is a simple but important part of the process. The therapist should ensure that the sandtray(s) and miniatures are in place. He or she should check to see that no miniatures are still buried in the sand from a previous session and should make sure that the sandtray surface is relatively flat and smooth. Furniture should be arranged so that the client(s) have easy access to the materials. The therapist should sit in a nonintrusive place in the room.

The introduction of the sandtray process may be directive or nondirective, depending on the therapeutic intent. The client can be invited to create any scene (or world, or picture) in the tray using the miniatures, or can be directed to make a specific scene around an event or emotion in the client's life or on a general or specific theme.

The creation of the tray is then left entirely up to the client. The therapist may do a number of things during the creation phase. This may include making no verbalizations to the client while providing full attendance to the client's work nonverbally. The therapist may choose to ask questions about the scene as it is unfolding, or may simply reflect the content of the building process much as a child-centered play therapist might do.

Some sandtray therapists prefer to let the creative process stand alone. While this is valuable, we believe that the process needs to be interactive and involve greater discussion. Thus, the creation serves as a springboard for discussion with the client.

The postcreation phase is a key aspect of the sandtray therapy process. Regardless of the initial instructions given to the client, it is still appropriate and necessary to discuss the tray with the client. Generally, clients are asked to give a title to the tray and to offer an explanation of the contents. As in narrative therapy, it is considered important for clients to tell their story, and the sandtray provides a nonverbal means through which to do this. Clients may be asked to describe the entire scene or portions of it or to discuss specific miniatures. They may be asked whether or not they themselves are represented in the tray or whether any other specific person is represented, and they are often asked what miniature(s) has (have) the greatest power in the tray.

It is important for the sandtray therapist to consider several things in the evaluation of the client's sandtray. These include an assessment of the creative process itself, the sandtray's contents, the client's story, and the therapist's own affective response to the tray. Here we would repeat our earlier warning against being too interpretive. Again, we wish to stress the importance of the clients' own interpretation of the therapeutic metaphors in their own creation.

The sandtray cleanup may be done within the session or after the client has left. This issue is generally left up to the client. Since the tray is an expression of the client's own emotional world, therapists are advised not to clean that world up without the client's direction and approval. It is also helpful to remind some clients that the tray and miniatures are used by others, and as such their tray cannot be preserved until the next session.

Documentation of the session should include the routine maintenance of client records, but also include a photograph or sketch of the client's tray. This provides a visual and chronological record of the therapy process, which can be shared with clients to facilitate discussion and progress review.

CASE EXAMPLES

Courtney, a 15-year-old 10th grader, and her mother had been in counseling for several sessions. Courtney was having difficulty at school and had begun several school refusal behaviors. Her mother was unable to understand her daughter's difficulties, remembering her own high school years as "perfect." Courtney had been unable to connect with her mother on this issue or express the depth of her distress at school.

A directive sandtray experience was planned to assist this mother–teen dyad about how to understand each other on a new level. The counselor began the session by dividing the sandtray into two parts by simply moving her hand through the sand. The clients were instructed to "build a scene in your half of the tray that expresses what your week has been like." Both clients began working easily and purposefully. Mother built a scene with a waterfall and pond, trees, and a house. She added three human figures in an equilateral triangle all looking straight ahead, not turned in for a relationship perspective. She later identified these as a mother, son, and daughter. Her husband did not appear in the tray. Courtney placed four fence sections in a square in the center of her half of the tray. In the center of the fenced-in area, she placed a small female teenage figure (Dorothy from the Wizard of Oz figures). On the outside of each piece of fence, facing inward toward the girl, was a T-Rex dinosaur. Courtney completed her part of the tray first and watched her mother finish.

Both the counselor and Courtney were very aware how self-absorbed the mother had become. Only upon saying that she was done did the mother glance at Courtney's scene. The shock of the contrast between her scene and her daughter's instantly registered on her face. Processing this tray allowed Courtney to finally verbalize that she felt all alone in trying to deal with overwhelming expectations (grades, popularity, "best time of her life," dating, etc.). Her mother was able to begin to understand that living in a "perfect" world was isolating her from both Courtney, her son, and her husband. This insight provided impetus for the mother to begin her own work in counseling.

In a case discussed in Homeyer and Sweeney (1998), the client was a 13-year-old boy who was referred for therapy after having been molested by two older boys in his neighborhood. He responded to his own sexual victimization by victimizing a younger foster girl in his home. His initial trays in therapy included multiple battle scenes—battles in which there were no victors. This was reflective of the client's emotional perception of his situation, which was indeed a place of great conflict from which he felt no escape. As the therapy continued, victories emerged from the battle, and provision was made for escape.

A very clear projection emerged in the sandtray scenes of this client, which involved scenes including the presence of two large figures, often a snake, alligator, or other large predatory animal. We have found it helpful to have a small number of such large predatory animal figures. When a client is exploring victimization issues in the tray, large predatory creatures are effective metaphors for the emotionally (and physically) overwhelming experiences of being victimized. Just as this client had been molested by two neighborhood adolescents, it was typical to see two large predatory creatures in most of his early trays. Later in the therapy process, he even named the two creatures with the same names as the offenders, information that was independently discovered by the therapist from the client's mother.

Later in the therapeutic process, the trays of this client showed a much greater degree of organization. The battle scenes were over, with this phase ending with a victor, which included the client himself. The greater order and freedom of the trays at the end of the process reflected a corresponding order and freedom in the client's life, reflected by decreased acting-out behaviors and emotional hypervigilance, and improved peer relations and school performance.

CONCLUSION

Sandtray therapy should focus on both the process and the product. An emphasis on one to the exclusion of the other deprives the client and the therapist of the full experience of therapeutic relationship. It is a spontaneous and dynamic process that brings clients to greater levels of awareness and appreciation of their own resources.

As with any expressive approach described in this book, it is important that persons wanting to do sandtray therapy get further training and supervised experience. This is a strong recommendation. It is also important for sandtray therapists to experience their own personal sandtray process. Jungian sandplay therapists place a very appropriate premium on helpers experiencing the process themselves. This is also a strong recommendation.

Sandtray therapy attracts therapists from a wide range of theoretical orientations. Use of the basic elements mentioned at the outset of this chapter can be adapted and adopted as effective tools for developing relationship and working through the process. Sandtray therapy carries the advantage of providing a nonverbal means of promoting healing, and is a process that values facilitation over direction, exploration over excavation, and growth over insight.

REFERENCES

Bowyer, L. R. (1970). *The Lowenfeld World Technique: Studies in personality.* New York: Pergamon Press.

Buhler, C. (1951a). The World Test: A projective technique. *Journal of Child Psychiatry, 2*(1), 4–23.

Buhler, C. (1951b). The World Test: Manual of directions. *Journal of Child Psychiatry, 2*(1), 69–81.

DeDomenico, G. (1995). *Sand tray world play: A comprehensive guide to the use of the sandtray in psychotherapeutic and transformational settings.* Oakland, CA: Vision Quest Images.

DeDomenico, G. (1999). Group sandtray-worldplay: New dimensions in sandplay therapy. In D. Sweeney & L. Homeyer (Eds.), *Handbook of group play therapy* (pp. 215–233). San Francisco: Jossey-Bass.

Erickson, E. (1951). Sex differences in the play configurations of pre-adolescents. *Journal of Orthopsychiatry, 21*, 667–692.

Harding (1947). Report on the Eighth Congress of Scandinavian Psychiatrists in Copenhagen, Denmark, 1946. *Acta Psychiatrica et Neurologica*, 294–314.

Homberger, E. (1938). Dramatic Production Test. In H. A. Murray (Ed.), *Explorations in personality* (pp. 558–582). New York: Oxford University Press.

Homeyer, L., & Sweeney, D. (1998). *Sandtray: A practical manual.* Canyon Lake, TX: Lindan Press.

Jones, L. (1983). The development of structure in the world of expression: A cognitive-developmental analysis of children's "sand worlds." *Dissertation Abstracts International, 43*(09B), 3052. (UMI No. 83–03178)

Kalff, D. (1980). *Sandplay: A psychotherapeutic approach to the psyche.* Santa Monica, CA: Sigo Press.

Lowenfeld, M. (1979). *The World Technique.* London: Allen & Unwin.

Lumry, G. (1951). Study of World Test characteristics as a basis for discrimination between various clinical categories. *Journal of Child Psychiatry, 2,* 24–35.

Mitchell, R. R., & Friedman, H. S. (1994). *Sandplay: Past, present and future.* London: Routledge.

Oaklander, V. (1988). *Windows to our children: A Gestalt therapy approach to children and adolescents.* Highland, NY: Center for Gestalt Development.

Oaklander, V. (1994). Gestalt play therapy. In K. O'Connor & C. Schaefer (Eds.), *Handbook of play therapy: Vol. 2. Advances and innovations* (pp. 143–156). New York: Wiley.

Petruk, L. (1996). *Creating a world in the sand: A pilot study of normative data for employing the sandtray as a diagnostic tool with children.* Unpublished master's thesis, Southwest Texas State University, San Marcos.

Schaefer, C. (1994). Play therapy for psychic trauma in children. In K. O'Connor & C. Schaefer (Eds.), *Handbook of play therapy: Vol. 2. Advances and innovations* (pp. 297–318). New York: Wiley.

Siegelman, E. Y. (1990). *Metaphor and meaning in psychotherapy.* New York: Guilford Press.

Sjolund, M. (1981). Play-diagnosis and therapy in Sweden: The Erica-Method. *Journal of Clinical Psychology, 37*(2), 322–325.

Sjolund, M. (1993). *The ERICA method: A technique for play therapy and diagnosis: A training guide.* Greeley, CO: Carron Publishers.

Stevens, R. (1983). *Erik Erikson: An introduction.* New York: St. Martin's Press.

Weinrib, E. (1983). *Images of self: The sandplay therapy process.* Boston: Sigo Press.

Wells, H. G. (1911). *Floor games.* New York: Arno Press. (Originally published in England. First U.S. edition, 1912)

Expressive Therapy

An Integrated Arts Approach

KAREN ESTRELLA

Expressive therapy as a treatment modality is founded on the interrelatedness of the arts and takes an integrated approach to the use of the arts as a tool for psychotherapy. Also referred to as expressive arts therapy, integrative arts therapy, multimodal expressive therapy, or intermodal expressive therapy, this approach represents a discipline rooted in philosophical, cultural/historical, and clinical models that each support the unique contributions that an interdisciplinary approach to the arts affords. Expressive therapists use a multimodal approach—at times working with the arts in sequence, at other times using the arts simultaneously, and at still other times carefully transitioning from one art form to another within the therapeutic encounter. Practitioners are trained to be sensitive to the unique properties within each art form, to be attentive to the creative process as a method of inquiry, and to be skilled at the integration of the arts, at times through a process known as the *intermodal transfer* (Knill, 1978).

The purpose of this chapter is to review the history of expressive arts therapy, describe the work of several leading theorists, and present clinical examples to illustrate this approach.

HISTORY

As the newest of the creative arts therapy disciplines, expressive therapy found its first clear articulation in the United States in a community of therapists, artists, scholars, and students at the Lesley College Graduate School's Institute for the Arts and Human Development in the1970s in Cambridge, Massachusetts (Levine & Levine, 1999). This integrated arts approach began as a collaborative project by core and adjunct faculty. The 1960s and 1970s were an era of experimentation, not only in therapy and education, but also in the arts. The multimedia and performance art movements of the time were just as influential as the human potential movements in challenging conventional boundaries to self-expression and artistic expression (Fleshman & Fryrear, 1981). The early artist-therapists at Lesley were interested in superseding their disciplinary divisions and realizing the untapped potential for the use of the arts in community, therapy, and education.

As this interdisciplinary approach became more established, these early innovators began to write about the roots of their work in philosophy, cultural theory, aesthetics, psychological theories, and clinical practice. As early as 1978, Paolo Knill had written a monograph on *Intermodal Learning in Education and Therapy,* which was used as required reading for students in the Lesley program. (This work would not see its entry into a more public domain until Knill, 1994, and then as a text coauthored with Helen Barba and Margot Fuchs [Knill, Barba, & Fuchs, 1995].) By 1981, other writers had acknowledged the purposeful use of an interdisciplinary approach to the arts as therapy (Fleshman & Fryrear, 1981; McNiff, 1981; Naitove, 1980). The most prominent example of this writing was McNiff's (1981) groundbreaking book, *The Arts and Psychotherapy.* In this text, he explored the historical, aesthetic, and philosophical applications of the arts to psychotherapy, and explored the use of the arts as inquiry and as psychotherapeutic encounter. (It is still used today in training programs in the expressive therapies.)

At the same time, debates about the legitimacy of the approach surfaced (Agell, 1982; Levick, 1980; McNiff, 1982; Naitove, 1980). These debates focused on the tension between generalists and specialists. Were expressive arts therapists sufficiently grounded in the arts, and if so, how could they demonstrate competence in all artistic media? Were they "jacks of all trades" and masters of none? Was there a discipline that could be mastered in this integrative approach? Upon what theoretical foundation did these newest creative arts therapists rely? Was the work of expressive therapists merely a "flirtation" with each of the more established individual arts therapies, such as music therapy, art therapy, and dance therapy?

These debates left their mark on expressive therapists' struggle to create a professional identity. Despite the establishment of the National Coalition of Arts Therapies Associations (NCATA) in 1979 (an alliance of six creative arts therapies associations: art therapy, dance therapy, music therapy, psychodrama, drama therapy, and poetry therapy), there was limited communication and cooperation between these individual arts therapy disciplines. Instead, each association evolved in a "dynamic and creative manner," utilizing its resources to establish itself more definitively (McNiff, 1986, p. 4). This commitment to specialization, however, left a professional gap for expressive arts therapists, who did not consider their work to be the mastery of each specialization, but who rather believed it to be the mastery of the principles of integration and wholeness that underlie the specializations (Levine, 1992). Several called for unification of the associations into one National Creative Arts Therapies Association (Naitove, 1980; Johnson, 1984, 1999; McNiff, 1986, 1987) in which a respect for "both specialized and integrated uses of media" could be established (McNiff, 1987, p. 271). This vision for the creative arts therapies, however, has yet to be realized in North America.

By contrast, our European counterparts have achieved some unified professional structures—for example, in 1991 the European Consortium for Arts Therapies Education (ECArTE) was founded. It now has 27 member institutions from 10 European countries (*www.uni-muenster.de/ Ecarte/*). However, an integrated approach to the arts is still not acknowledged as a separate discipline even within this consortium; instead art therapy, dance therapy, drama therapy, and music therapy are specified. In the Netherlands, however, as early as the late 1950s and 1960s a new form of "creative therapy" was developed, a therapy that included several media, but was grounded in the concept of change that arises out of unblocked creativity. The Dutch Association for Creative Therapy (Nederlandse Vereniging voor Creatieve Therapie) currently oversees creative arts therapies in the Netherlands (for a more complete description and history, see McNiff, 1986, 1987; see also Smerijsters, 1993). Another example in Europe throughout the 1980s was Phillip Speiser's coordination of an integrated arts therapy approach in Sweden and Scandinavia (Speiser, 1996).

The exclusion of expressive therapy as an integrative arts approach in NCATA or ECArTE has resulted from both the discipline's ambivalence with establishing itself as yet another distinct "specialization" and from early splits among expressive therapists themselves. Pioneers in the field of expressive therapy have been reluctant to form yet another "brand" of creative arts therapy, favoring instead the inclusion of a multidisciplinary approach by all creative arts therapies (McNiff, 1986, 2000). The hope was that the existing specializations would each recognize the value in providing both specialized *and* integrated uses of the arts as a tool for therapy, rather than expressive therapists using valuable energy and resources on developing further credentials, educational requirements, and professional associations. Many wished that the individual arts associations would form a larger alliance, not for the sake of "fusing" the arts therapies, as Johnson (1985) states, but rather for the sake of strengthening the common ground upon which each of the creative arts therapies stand—the ground of creative expression, body–mind–soul integration, and aesthetic experience.

One of the main obstacles to both unification and inclusion of an integrated approach to the arts proved to be that each creative arts therapy specialization was "both defined and divided by [their] allegiance to [their] particular art media" (Johnson, 1985, p. 234). Expressive therapists have been reluctant to join this "allegiance" to specialization by further defining themselves, especially in terms of their relation to the media of the arts. Nonetheless, some central ideas have emerged from this integrative approach that can provide coherence. I will expand upon these, but first I would like to comment on some common factors among the creative arts therapies.

THE LINK AMONG THE
CREATIVE ARTS THERAPIES

Over the years a body of knowledge has emerged that recognizes the "link among the creative arts therapies" (Johnson, 1985) and that bases itself on "shared qualities" such as "action, the use of arts media, nonverbal expression, a commitment to creative transformation, etc." (McNiff, 1987, p. 272). These links, and this action orientation, have come to be recognized by more mainstream oganizations and mental health constituencies, as evidenced by two edited volumes on the use of expressive techniques in therapy by the American Psychological Association (Wiener, 1999; Wiener & Oxford, 2003). While it is beyond the scope of this chapter to review all of this emerging body of literature, I would like to discuss some basic concepts. (The interested reader is referred to the excellent "Selected Bibliography on the Creative Arts Therapies"[Johnson, 1999, pp. 189–193], which divides these readings into books and journal articles, subdivided into professional, clinical, and theoretical categories.)

Given our diversity in technique, theory, and media, Johnson (1985) notes that, as creative arts therapists, we do better to define our common ground in a "basic perspective on the human condition, such as creativity, play, or aesthetic knowing" (p. 234). While our common ground may not lie in specific media-related concepts, there is much that underlies the creative arts therapies that is not media-based, but rather related to sensory-based expression, aesthetics, and the creative process itself. Expressive therapists have relied, in part, on these ideas as a basis for their work in the same way that integrative psychotherapists have relied on common curative factors among the various schools of psychotherapy (Lampropoulos, 2000). Expressive therapists study these common factors, and utilize them in making decisions about how to introduce and integrate the arts in their sessions.

Sensory-Based Expression

In his article "Envisioning the Link among the Creative Arts Therapies," Johnson (1985) describes one of our common strengths as our ability to utilize processes that rely on nonverbal, nondiscursive expressions (see also Robbins, 1980). The arts are uniquely beneficial in their capacity to access experience, thoughts, and feelings that do not depend exclusively on either verbal language or narrative discourse. This is not to say that art-based communication is exclusively nonverbal, but rather that by relying on sensory-based, image-based expression the arts have something unique to offer. Nonverbal approaches are also significant in that they provide particularly useful treatment for clients for whom verbal language is inaccessible (e.g., persons with aphasia or Alzheimer's disease). Also, these sensory/image-based communications may be potentially useful for those who have experienced trauma. In recent years, researchers have discovered that traumatic memories are not organized via a narrative, and that traumatized individuals are initially unable to arrange these memories in words or symbols. Instead, these traumatic memories are stored as somatic sensations, emotional vulnerabilities, flashbacks and nightmares, dissociative inclinations, and behavioral reenactments (Allen, 1993; van der Kolk & van der Hart, 1991).

As psychology becomes more interested in the mechanisms of affective engagement and affect regulation (Weston, 1994), the creative arts therapies have unique contributions to offer in the treatment of individuals who experience trouble with these processes. The creative arts therapies involve action. The concretization of image, symbol, relationship, and affect in artistic form offers "explicitness of the symbolic representation of emotionally-laden ideas" (Blatner, 1992, p. 406). The links between somatic experience and affective knowing, which psychologists are now unraveling, have long been intuited, and utilized, by creative arts therapists who recognize the unique ways that arts making engages affective, cognitive, and somatic processes simultaneously (see Johnson, 1987).

Aesthetics

Reliance upon the principles of aesthetics provides another common link among creative arts therapies. Aesthetics is the study of concepts such as "beauty, harmony, rhythm, resonance, brilliance, dynamic tension, and balance" (Johnson, 1985, p. 236)—clearly all qualities shared by artistic endeavors in or outside of therapy. The arts' capacity to give symbolic form to feelings lies at the heart of Langer's (1953) philosophy of aesthetics, and underlies much of creative arts therapy's reliance on her philosophy. The arts' ability to transcend individual experience and speak to and for our spiritually bereft, suffering soul also represents an aspect of aesthetic experience. As Levine and Levine (1999) assert, "the therapeutic power of art rests not in its elimination of suffering but rather in its capacity to hold us in the midst of that suffering so that we can bear the chaos without denial or flight" (p. 31).

Robbins (1985, 1988), who has perhaps been the most prolific theorist in this area, describes the development of aesthetic communication:

> Developmentally, from birth we struggle to transform our sensations and affects into symbolic form. This symbolization process, commonly called secondary process, becomes the basic glue in developing a self that maintains connections with the past, present and future. As we experience the inevitable developmental process of growth, we heal our splits, integrate opposites into symbolic form and work towards individualization. When symbolic form includes multiple levels of communication and becomes larger and more meaningful than its individual parts, we approach levels of aesthetic communication. (1985, pp. 67–68)

Several other writers who emphasize the common links among creative arts therapists also speak of this integrative function of aesthetics. Aldridge, Brandt, and Wohler (1990) note that

> the continuing therapeutic process is to give articulation to a broad range of human feelings . . . the escape from emotive fragmentation to the creative act of becoming whole. Our inner lives in all their depth and richness are given coherence and presented externally as created form. (p. 195)

Grenadier (1995) writes: "Our very faith in the art we practice is based upon a belief that psychic life is imaginal; that imagination is the larger container that bridges subject and object, holding and encompassing duality and psychic splits" (p. 400). For Grenadier, imagination is what lies between experience and meaning, the personal and the collective. It is this sense of value in aesthetics that is crucial to expressive therapists.

Creativity

Lastly, the creative process lies at the root of all creative arts therapies, and is fundamental in apprehending the integrated expressive arts approach. "There is a clear, definitive and common identity for all the creative arts therapies that centers on the *primary* use of creativity as a process of therapeutic transformation" (McNiff, 1986, p. 15). It is essential that integrative arts therapists understand theories of creativity, stages of creativity, and the unique "transformational urge" (Johnson, 1985) that creativity embodies. Along with an interest in Jungian depth psychology and the central ideas of active imagination (see McNiff's 1998 review of Joan Chodorow's work on Jung), Winnicott's theory of creativity has been of particular interest to creative arts therapists and integrated expressive arts therapists (S. K. Levine, 1992; E. Levine, 1995).

For Winnicott (1971), creativity ("primary creativity") is a basic human activity beginning with the infant's subjective experience, with "the illusion that there is an external reality [which] corresponds to the infant's own capacity to create" (p. 12). Winnicott believes that the function of illusion is to mediate subjective experience with objective reality via the *potential space*, which he proposes takes place originally between the primary caretaker and the infant, but later throughout life. This infantile ability to create illusion and to construct mental representations is the building block of intersubjective experience and relational knowing, and is central to the initial formations of a self-identity and of social cognition. Our involvement in the mediation between subjective experience and objective reality lays the foundation for a tolerance of the dialogical nature of life. "What Winnicott is saying, implicitly, is that psychic life is imaginal; we live in the imaginative and playful space of experience" where the "boundary between interpretation and play would itself be permeable and shifting" (S. K. Levine, 1992, pp. 32–33). It is this experience of creativity and imagination in the transitional space that creative arts therapists re-create in their sessions—"that is, an aesthetic, imaginal, metaphoric space in which inside and outside, self and other, are mixed" (Johnson, 1998, p. 89).

The last aspect of creativity I would like to discuss is the stages of creativity. Understanding the stages of the creative process is important in understanding our clients' use of the arts. Goren-Bar (1997) describes the process of creativity through his six-stage "creation axis" model. This model provides the expressive arts therapist a way of reconstructing and reporting about his or her client's creative process, a means of understanding the clinical relevance of the creative process at various stages, and options for intervening during the creative process (Goren-Bar, 1997, p. 411).

In the first phase, the *organizational phase*, the first three stages—(1) contact, (2) organization, and (3) improvisation—imply the "how" of what the client creates. What is the client's level of curiosity? How does he or she contact with and organize the artistic materials and his or her relationship to them? What is his or her skill and how does he or she approach problem solving with the materials? How flexible and spontaneous is he or she? How responsive to the materials is he or she? In the second phase, the *content-symbolic phase*, the last three stages—(4) central theme, (5) elaboration (variation), and (6) preservation—are concerned primarily with "what" the client represents in symbolic form, the content that absorbs the client. What are the central themes in which the client chooses to invest? Now that a certain mastery has been achieved, how does the client elaborate on his or her theme? What is the process by which he or she lets go of his or her piece? How is the artwork preserved or presented? What life does the artwork take on separate from the client? Goren-Bar offers us a model that makes the creative process explicit. He offers specific clinical criteria linked to the creative process with which one can communicate with colleagues who have not been trained in expressive therapy, and from which one can assess and intervene with clients.

Given the centrality of the creative process in creative arts therapy practice, we are obligated to develop models that look specifically at the mechanisms of change initiated by the therapeutic process in the arts. Johnson (1998) has developed such a model, and I would encourage readers to look more closely at his specific model of the "therapeutic action of the creative arts therapies." Building on psychodynamic theory, Johnson looks specifically at the processes of projection of internalized and externalized self-objects, transformation, and internalization as they specifically relate to artistic expression and the arts/playspace in the context of creative arts therapies.

There is much to be gained by examining the common ground of creative arts therapies. The use of sensory-based expression, aesthetic principles, and creativity are but a few of the commonalities shared among creative arts therapies. Expressive arts therapists are interested in the unique contributions of each modality as well as the common factors that underlie our professions. Integrated arts therapists have often utilized this literature, which articulates the links among the arts therapies, in favor of creating new theories and models of their own. Yet, despite this, a growing body of literature specific to expressive arts therapy theory is emerging.

CREATING A DISTINCT SPECIALIZATION

In the last few years, expressive therapists have taken up the task of defining themselves as a distinct discipline (Speiser, 1996). The emergence of the International Expressive Arts Therapy Association (IEATA) in 1994 came as a result of a split among expressive therapists over professional affiliation and organizational structure. Many members of IEATA were originally members of the American Association of Artists-Therapists, founded in 1978. The American Association of Artists-Therapists was grounded in an all-inclusive "reconceptualization of therapy to include artistic process as a primary component" (Speiser, 1996, p. 78). In the late 1980s, this organization changed its name, first to the American Expressive Therapy Association, and then to the National Expressive Therapy Association, and entered into rancorous conflict with other creative arts therapy specializations. One result of these divisions was the development of IEATA, but perhaps another by-product was the continued isolation of the discipline of expressive therapy from the other creative arts therapies. Since its inception, IEATA has become the professional home for many integrative arts therapists. Once again, expressive arts therapy has begun the process of legitimizing standard professional practice of expressive arts therapy via a registration process for expressive arts therapists and seeking cooperation with other creative arts therapy associations (see *www.ieata.org*).[1]

In addition to the development of a new democratic association, several texts specific to integrative work have been published since the early 1990s (Atkins, 2002; Knill et al., 1995; E. Levine, 1995; S. K. Levine, 1992; Levine & Levine, 1999; Rogers, 1993). Knill et al. (1995) note that "intermodal expressive therapy *is a discipline unto itself,* with its own theoretical framework and focus" (emphasis in original, p. 16). In their "Foundations of Expressive Arts Therapy," Levine and Levine (1999) claim that expressive arts therapists are "specialists in intermodality; that is, . . . capable of grasping the junctures at which one mode of artistic expression needs to give way to, or be supplemented by, another" (p. 11). It is this "specialization in intermodality" that I wish to further illuminate in this chapter.

Before I begin, however, I would like to note the paradox of trying to *define* a "specialization in intermodality." The very nature of the integrative approach is founded upon an opening up of possibilities of expression, not a delimiting of experience. While I will try to explicate some theoretical principles of an integrated arts therapy, these ideas are in no way meant to be the definitive unification of a theory of expressive arts therapy. Levine and Levine (1999) pose the question of whether a single theoretical framework for expressive therapy is possible or even desirable. They note that it is the very diversity and multiplicity of theoretical frameworks and practical approaches that gives expressive therapy its life. Yet like Johnson's call to the creative arts therapies, I feel that unless we as expressive therapists are to be "more than a valued decoration on the great edifice of modern psychiatry" (or even on the emerging edifice of creative arts therapies), "we must be able to articulate our unique contributions . . . differentiate a wide range of professional roles

---

[1]While IEATA's registration of expressive arts therapists (REAT) is most widely respected (see *www.ieata.org/IEATA%20Standards.html*), the National Expressive Therapy Association (NETA) also has a certification process. IEATA registers only master's-level clinicians. NETA, on the other hand, makes a distinction between "expressive arts therapy" and "expressive therapy," certifying both bachelor's-level and master's-level individuals with minimal expressive therapy training (See *www.expressivetherapy.com/htmls/standards.html*).

within our profession . . . [and] provide the conditions for mature leadership" (Johnson, 1984, p. 209).

MAJOR APPROACHES

Knill's Intermodal Theory

Knill's theory of intermodal expressive therapy developed as a natural extension of his background as a performance artist and his interest in polyaesthetics (an interdisciplinary method, designed in the 1950s by Wolfgang Roscher, for teaching the arts). Knill et al. (1995) advocate for a "specialization in the interdisciplinary tradition of the arts" that performance-based arts exemplify (p. 17). Central to the theory of polyaesthetics is the idea that all of the sensory and communicative modalities exist within each art form—so that within music, for example, lies the rhythm of dance; the structure, form, and color of art; the phrasing and lyricism of poetry; and the motifs and stories of dramatic enactment (Knill et al., 1995, p. 28). Each art form contains within it the seeds of the other arts through aesthetics and sensory perception. It is this quality that makes the media of television, advertising, and film so powerful. Commercials have long exploited the power of polyaesthetics by combining music, dramatic enactment, and visual aesthetics in the marketing of their products. These continuities among the arts are intuitively experienced and provide a means by which communication can be enhanced across arts-based expression.

In addition, Knill et al. (1995) note that psychic material naturally strives for "optimal clarity and precision of feeling and thought" via a process they call *crystallization* (p. 30).

> The metaphor of crystallization is used to explain how in an environment saturated with artistic imagination, a small creative act, seen as a seed, will grow. The growth, then following ancient traditions of the arts, reveals the seed's full meaning with the clarity and order of a crystal. (Knill, 1994, p. 322)

Within the triangular relationship of client, artwork/art process, and therapist, an attempt is made to facilitate meaning making in the context of the imaginative process via the "language of the imagination" (Knill, 1994, p. 322). It is this therapeutic relationship created via the imaginative realm that "provides optimal conditions for emerging images to disclose their meanings through the use of different arts disciplines" (Knill, 1994, p. 322). By paying attention to the interpersonal, intrapersonal, and transpersonal functions of the arts in the experience, one can facilitate an expression that is "optimally clear and understandable"(Knill et al., 1995, p. 150); these functions include centering and individuation, expression and catharsis, containment and documentation, meaning and sense making, and communication and communion (Knill et al., 1995, pp. 46–55).

It is these two principles, polyaesthetics and crystallization theory, that make the intermodal process quite clear (Knill, 1994). Intermodal theory rests on the process of the *intermodal transfer* and the *intermodal superimposition.* The intermodal transfer involves shifting from one art form to another (Knill et al., 1995, p. 36). Intermodal superimposition involves the adding on of art forms in order to "amplify the imagination" (p. 151). Likening this process to Gendlin's (1981) process of focusing, Knill et al. note that by identifying the corresponding aesthetic elements within an artistic expression, the therapist invites the client to augment his or her expression with the goal of revealing the "quite right" image (Knill et al., 1995, p. 36). By asking the client, for example, to find the corresponding gesture to his or her rhythm or sound for his or her painting, or story for his or her movement, the therapist invites the client to amplify, clarify, or emotionally accentuate his or her original expression, whether this is a verbal description or a first attempt at artistic examination. It is this "grasping the junctures at which one mode of artistic expression needs to give way to, or be supplemented by, another" that the intermodalist is striving to facilitate (Levine & Levine, 1999, p. 11).

But how is the therapist to know when to suggest a transfer? What are the clinical indications that an intermodal transfer, or superimposition, is called for? When is an intermodal transfer inadvisable? Knill et al. (1995) suggest that intermodal expressive therapists demonstrate a committed presence within the session, approaching the client's expression with a "low skill-high sensitivity" approach (p. 149). By paying particular attention to facilitating an arts-based experience that is accessible, regardless of the client's art experience or training, the therapist stays sensitive to the ways in which the expression can more clearly express the client's intention.

When considering the suitability of an intermodal transfer or superimposition, the therapist uses the interpersonal, intrapersonal, and transpersonal functions of the arts expression to assess the appropriate intervention. For example, one might ask: Is individuation or socialization being emphasized in this session, and which art media will enhance that process? Which arts processes will best facilitate the need to distance from this psychological material or to engage it more fully? This ability of the therapist to recognize the degree of emotional distance or disclosure involved in an artistic modality or expression is one of the common principles that underlie the creative arts therapies (Blatner, 1992). As the intermodal therapist becomes more familiar with the elements of each of the various art forms, he or she is able to recognize the properties that these elements elicit—so that, for example, collaborative music making may enhance socialization, while individual painting may enhance introspection.

Another consideration for intermodal work is the comfort level of the client with a particular modality. Knill et al. (1995) suggest that we "develop a sensitivity to people's literal or imagined barriers to engaging the various modalities," and begin where people are most comfortable (p. 146). They suggest that we stay mindful of introducing a "threatening" modality that might inhibit the expressing person (p. 152). This is similar to Goren-Bar's (1994) admonishment to pay attention to the client's "home land," or dominant modality (p. 58). Goren-Bar (1994) warns against premature transfers. He recommends that intermodal transfers not be suggested before clients have "explored and fully experienced the modality with which they have begun work," and, as such, he proposes that transfers be avoided during the first three stages of his creation-axis model (p. 58). Knill et al. (1995) also warn against too rapid a pace because this can interfere with the therapeutic and creative process. Lastly, they recommend that the therapist guard against choosing a modality that does not allow for the continuation of the experience, being mindful not to take the individual or the group too far away from his, her, or their original expression or intention (p. 152).

McNiff's Theory of Art as Medicine

Shaun McNiff's commitment to an integrative approach to the arts is rooted in his belief that "art by its nature includes everything imaginable" (McNiff, 1982, p. 123). All of the elements of creative expression—imagery, sound, gesture, words, enactment, movement—work together, all are aspects of the human imagination and cannot be separated, either in art or in life (McNiff, 1982). McNiff (1986) believes that the creative arts therapies have a unique contribution to make in a society that is bereft of cultural and spiritual connections and roots, and that is in dire need of "the restoration of an ancient and archetypal integration of the creative process with healing" (p. 5). For McNiff, "a primal and unspoken spiritual motive" lies beneath the rise of the creative arts therapies. The arts provide soul medicine, and McNiff (1992) proposes that we conceptualize arts therapy as a "therapy of the imagination."

McNiff is less interested in specific techniques of intermodal process and more interested in "the successful activation of creative 'energy' "— "a primary objective of my practice has been the creation of a space that generates expressive energies which then act upon the people within it" (McNiff, 2000, p. 320). McNiff's unwavering commitment to, and trust and belief in, the healing properties of the creative process underlie all his work. Central to this belief is a deep respect for the imaginal realm. McNiff has long advocated that the powers of imagination not take second place within the creative arts therapies to psychological theories or cognitive framing of creative experience. Instead, he has proposed that we develop a theory indigenous to art, an artistic psychology, in which the mode of psychological inquiry is artistic expression and reflection (McNiff, 1992).

McNiff (1988) has grounded his theory in "ancient continuities in art, health, and religion" (p. 285). His embrace of the archetype of the shaman dates back to 1979, when he published his first article on this subject, "From Shamanism to Art Therapy" (see McNiff, 1979).

> If we look to the past and to the healing practices of indigenous cultures, there is considerable evidence that creative expression and healing belong together. In these traditions the religious and philosophical consciousness is integrated with what might be described as more "scientifically" oriented healing practices. (McNiff, 1986, p. 6)

By bringing their awareness to this interplay, many creative arts therapists draw on the interrelatedness of the arts, religion, healing, and cultural practices, thereby allowing the client, via a "sacred" approach to the arts and healing, to bring his or her whole self—body, mind, emotions, spirit, and soul—to recovery. McNiff's approach rejects modern psychology's fundamental reliance on rationalism, its disconnection from soul work, and its embrace of interventions that serve to further depersonalize the "patient" (e.g., an overreliance on psychopharmacology). Instead, he proposes that by active engagement in the imaginative realm, "the transformative and healing powers of the psyche" are released (McNiff, 1986, p. 9; see also McNiff, 1992).

McNiff advocates that the imaginal realm be activated by the invitation to engage in multiple forms of art making. This art making can take place with individuals, in small groups, or in large groups. An example of the creation of this imaginal realm can be seen in McNiff's (2000) description of his arts studio group work. Having the members of the group move freely, in a relaxed way, to live drumming creates an atmosphere of spontaneity and improvisation. Members approach their painting and drawing as movement. Elemental gestures become the basis for markings in art, and the continued presence of music and sound while painting allows the members "to let go and move more spontaneously in their painting . . . energizing the painting process" (p. 323).

McNiff trusts the psyche, once engaged, to make itself known, via the imagination and the arts. The images and expressions that emerge in this environment become the messengers of healing. A multimodal approach can then be used in reflecting upon the image, in the same way that it was used in creating it. McNiff proposes that by further imagining the image, we can "amplify and focus our engagement" with it (McNiff, 2000, p. 321). In order to maximize our engagement with the image, McNiff (1992) suggests that we view our images as "co-participants" in the inquiry process (p. 63). By establishing the "otherness" of the image, the potential for dialogue and interplay are activated. Building on Jung's process of "active imagination," McNiff suggests dialoguing with our images. By entering the imaginal realm, figures within the image (and even nonfigural aspects of the image such as color or texture), or the image as a whole, is given voice and allowed to speak its truth (McNiff, 1992, p. 84). By allowing ourselves to become further engaged in the image—by taking on the role of some aspect of the image—we perpetuate the imaginal realm and the potential for healing within it.

McNiff (1992) suggests creating the "creation story" of an image, talking with and to one's image, using "movement, dramatic action, voice, sounds, and changes in personal appearance and the environment" to "become physically incorporated into the imagination of the painting" via performance art, as all possible ways of further imagining the image (p. 119). In recent years, in a desire to break free of the restrictions of the "linear structure of narrative," McNiff (2000) has become even more interested in the use of movement, vocal expression, and performance as a means of accessing "the creative energies manifested by image" (p. 321). These return him to an ongoing theme throughout his work: that "transformative therapeutic engagement occurs within the primary language of the image, the body, and physical enactment" (McNiff, 1986, p. 9).

Rogers's Creative Connection

Natalie Rogers has developed a model of expressive therapy grounded in the person-centered approach developed by her father, Carl Rogers. Founded on the principles of empathy, congruence, and unconditional positive regard, which characterize the person-centered philosophy, Rogers's model focuses upon the facilitating environment created by the therapist's commitment to the individual's "trustworthy" movement toward self-realization and growth. Rogers elaborates on her father's approach by recognizing that people have "a need to fulfill their creative capacities. An inherent impulse or drive within each of us longs for creative expression" (Rogers, 1993, p. 96). It is in response to this "inherent impulse" that Rogers has developed the Creative Connection process, a process based on "the enhancing interplay among movement, art, writing, and sound" (p. 4).

Given our culture's predisposition to verbalization, Rogers prescribes "carefully planned experiments or experiences" that "would motivate and allow people time and space to engage in the creative process" (p. 17). As with Knill's model, Rogers suggests allowing clients to begin their art making in safe, comfortable, nonjudgmental ways. Like McNiff, she feels that our society has forgotten its roots of creativity and healing, and that people need to be reminded of their basic needs for creative expression. She elaborates on the frequent experience our clients have of blocks to their creativity, and emphasizes the need to engage creativity in an environment free of judgment, fear, and criticism.

In her book *The Creative Connection*, Rogers (1993) offers exercises designed to promote client access to creativity, self-awareness, and self-empowerment. For example, as a beginning exploration, Rogers suggests an experiment she calls "The Big Doodle" (p. 28). The participant begins by choosing a color marker, closing his or her eyes, and singing or humming to him- or herself. The participant is encouraged to begin by making big doodles in the air, allowing his or her arms to dance, then making doodles on paper, humming and singing all the while, inviting him- or herself to be playful and have fun. The participant is encouraged to make several doodles, as many as needed to "satisfy your playful urge." Once completed, one or two doodles that are particularly appealing to the client are selected for further elaboration—first in art, then in writing, and finally as a springboard to movement or sound. Rogers suggests "dancing the picture" and allowing sounds to emerge from the dance. This exercise is a designed as a method of practicing nonjudgment, of allowing creativity to emerge and to spiral into a process of self-exploration.

This process of moving from one art form to another, of superimposing one art form with another, lies at the heart of Rogers's method of the Creative Connection.

> By moving from art form to art form, we release layers of inhibition that have covered our originality, discovering our uniqueness and special beauty. Like a spiral, the process plumbs the depths of our body, mind, emotions, and spirit to bring us to our center. This center or core is our essence, our wellspring of creative vitality. (Rogers, 1993, p. 43)

Rogers suggests this transition from one art form to another as a means of heightening and intensifying "our journey inward" (p. 43). Through contact with our center we are opened up to "the universal energy source, bringing us vitality and a sense of oneness" (p. 44). In addition to the active forms of the creative process, Rogers also emphasizes the importance of meditation and receptive forms of creativity (p. 50).

Rogers encourages the therapist to listen to the client's language for clues—if the client uses visual words as descriptors, for example, the therapist may begin with art; if the client is using movement words, then the therapist may begin with movement. A feeling, an image, a concept or metaphor, or a bodily impulse can each be used as inspiration for creative action. If the client was speaking of how powerless he or she feels, this concept of "powerlessness" can become a springboard for creative expression: What would this powerlessness look like? Sound like? How does powerless feel in your body? What shape would it take? As the client is able to trust the environment to be free from judgment, he or she too becomes free to trust and respect his or her inner world. Rogers takes a strong process-oriented approach, emphasizing that interpretations of the meaning of the art stay client-centered. She is strongly opposed to analyzing client's creative expressions, and insists that therapists follow the lead of the client, leaving the authority, decision-making, and meaning-making processes with the client (p. 102).

Lusebrink's Expressive Therapy Continuum

The last model I would like to introduce is not a model of expressive therapy per se, but it does have much relevance for expressive arts therapists in that it provides us with a developmental model of creative expression from which we can assess, plan, and intervene. Lusebrink's (1992) Expressive Therapy Continuum (ETC) is a three-level, hierarchical, developmental model, based on a sequence of "increased complexity in cognitive and emotional development" (p. 395). This model describes clients' internal processes, their interaction with the artistic media, and their level of expression. The first level is the kinesthetic/sensory level, the second level is the perceptual/affective level, and the third level is the cognitive/symbolic level. "Creative expression can be manifested on any of the levels of the ETC," and can be seen as its own level made up of contributions from different components of the other levels (Lusebrink, 1992, p. 402). Each level has a "healing dimension," an aspect of the level that represents "optimum intrapersonal functioning" on that level; and an "emergent function," aspects of the level that develop "characteristics of the next higher level" (p. 395).

The sensory/kinesthetic level represents the client's most primal interactions with artistic media. Inner sensations, physical release of energy, spontaneous movement, and sensory involvement are all characteristic of this level. The two components of each level enhance and balance one another. Sensory awareness is given external expression in kinesthetic bodily response, and increased kinesthetic activity can raise awareness of sensate experience. In kind, the more attention is given to sensory awareness, the more slowed down the kinesthetic involvement, and vice versa. Rhythm acts as a basic organizing principle for people, and serves as one of the most basic healing dimensions of this level, along with energy release and awareness of inner sensation. As visceral, tactile, audio, or visual sensations and proprioceptive/kinesthetic movement form, "internal and external form perception, image formation and expression of affect" result, which constitute the emergent function of this level (Lusebrink, 1992, p. 398).

The perceptual/affective level is characterized by emotional expression, affective-based imagery, form perception, awareness of schemas, and awareness of the formal and structural qualities of imagery. Once again the two components enhance and balance one another. "The perceptual aspect gives form to emotions . . . the affective component, in turn, gives a dynamic quality to forms and endows them with personal qualities" (p. 399). On the other hand, too much emphasis on form can dampen the emotional quality, and too much emotion can distort form. The healing dimension of this level involves the organization of sensory-based stimuli (visual, auditory, and kinesthetic), the formation of perceptual Gestalts that work, and the appropriate channeling of affect. The emergent function of this level is "the interaction of schemes and the formation of symbolic affect" (p. 400).

The cognitive/symbolic level is characterized by problem-solving, decision-making, analytical, and reality-directed cognitive processes, as well as by metaphor and symbol formation, and the expression of symbolic imagery. "Symbols are multileveled and multidimensional and encompass kinesthetic, affective and the structural components" (p. 400). As emphasis is placed on the cognitive component of expression, the symbolic components are put into focused reality, and as emphasis is placed on the symbolic aspects of the expression, a more intuitive perspective is given to the problem-solving aspects of the expression. As such, an overemphasis on either the cognitive or the symbolic components can diminish the other's healing dimensions. The healing dimensions of this level involve the development and expression of personally significant symbols and the insight involved in these expressions. The emergent function of this level leads to "creative problem solving using verbal and imaginal integration, and to insight and the discovery of new or repressed parts of the self" (p. 402).

The Expressive Therapy Continuum provides a means of recognizing the developmental components of creative expression. Expressive therapists are able to assess the level of their client's involvement in the various components; for example, observations can be made of the client's involvement in the sensory component of expression or the affective component of expression. In addition, intermodal transfers, amplifications, or superimpositions can be made that can enhance or elicit various components or levels of expression. For instance, in the example of McNiff's studio work described earlier, the kinesthetic awareness of moving one's arms and of listening to the rhythm of the drumming is enhanced by the perceptual awareness of finding form in one's markings that correspond to one's movements. The Expressive Therapy Continuum provides expressive therapists with a way to conceptualize their client's movement across and within modalities.

CLINICAL APPLICATIONS

In this section, I describe three examples of expressive therapy in clinical practice. All identifying information has been changed to protect clients' confidentiality.

Expressive Therapy Group Work in Adult Day Treatment

Adults living with schizophrenia, manic–depressive illness, and chronic depression often lose relationships, community, and continuity with work and self-worth. For 5 years I worked as the expressive therapist at a day treatment program for adults diagnosed with major mental illnesses in an urban area. Our clients ranged in age from 18 to 80 and often remained in the program for several years. The primary treatment modality was group therapy. The expressive arts therapies were a large component of our program. Expressive therapy was particularly suitable as a treatment modality for the center's goals: revitalization of a sense of wellness, renewed self-esteem arising from interaction with others, integration of affect with cognitive and body-based tasks, and improved awareness of reality-based symptom management. Many of our groups centered on a theme or modality: family issues, art therapy, relaxation, songwriting, and so on. As the resident expressive therapist I utilized a multimodal approach to my groups.

In the songwriting group, for example, I often used art, movement, or drama to enhance the poetry and songwriting that provided a central focus. Each week the group explored themes relevant to the members, such as home, family, feelings, or self-worth. Members listened to songs with lyrics that contained the themes we were exploring and used the other modalities to enhance their personal connection or involvement with these themes. Members then created collective poems, which were set to music and performed for the larger community.

One example of an integrated arts process involved the creation of our version of the lyrics to Burt Bachrach and Hal David's "What the World Needs Now Is Love." The group began by listening to the song, and then identified a list of things or qualities they felt they each individually needed. As members shared their lists, the theme of "peace of mind" emerged. Over the next two meetings, the group explored the theme of "peace of mind." First, through guided imagery, each member was directed to envision him- or herself in a peaceful place. Next, each member wrote about his or her inner journey and experience. Members were then invited to represent their peaceful place in imagery by drawing or creating a collage. As the representations of what each member needed became solidified, their collective experience took shape in a poem, which was used as our revised lyrics to the song:

Chorus:
What we all need now is peace of mind
It's the only way to leave our pain behind
What we all need now is peace of mind
We could just relax and we'd all be fine

Lord we don't need more war or failures
We don't need to be reminded of mistakes we've made
We don't need confrontations or conflicts, no
Or cancer, no—we don't want to fade (chorus)

What some of us need is love and money
We need music and dancing and happiness
We need a job and a car and lots of health
And harmony, and we need it soon (chorus)

Group pride was evident as each member proudly sang along when we shared our joint creations with the larger community. Our creative expressions allowed members to give voice to their struggles in handling the losses and the impact on their self-esteem that came with being diagnosed with a major mental illness. A revived sense of hope came from envisioning a better, more peaceful place for themselves and each other.

Expressive Therapy Group Work with Court-Involved Adolescents

The teenage girls I worked with in an inner-city detention center were just as much in need of the arts as a tool for self-expression and transformation as the adults in day treatment. Ironically, without any awareness of themselves as multimodal artists, the girls lived lives filled with the arts. As teenagers living in a hip-hop culture, they saw music, dance, language, art, and dress as pieces of the whole. For these *girlz*, the arts represented their community and experience in a way that was already integrated in their lives. Yet their voices, their involvement in creating art, tended to be silenced in favor of a passive approach to the arts. Inviting them to create poetry, art, music, and dance became a source of empowerment for them, a means for their voices to be heard, for their needs to be articulated. This was easier done when the arts corresponded to the arts with which they were most familiar, and when initiated by responding to art. Beginning with artists they knew and respected was important. 2Pac, or Tupac Shakur (1995), explores the themes of grief, gratitude, loss, fear, violence, sex, honesty, loyalty, betrayal, prison, and family—themes with which many of the girls struggled to come to terms.

2Pac's music became our springboard for an intermodal process lasting several weeks. His song, "Shed So Many Tears" is about loss, gang warfare, teenage pregnancy, and death. After listening to the song, girls wrote their reactions. Pictures of graveyards and descriptions of friends they had known who had died emerged spontaneously. These reactions became the basis for our own version of "The DYS [Department of Youth Services] Blues." Maria, a small, quiet, angry, 15-year-old girl from the Dominican Republic, was particularly moved as she wrote about being bounced in and out of foster homes and the death of her brother in gang warfare. The girls were vulnerable and grieving as we explored these issues. Where was their protection? What advice could they take with them? Maria suggested that we make "guardian angels." We had previously made small sculpture figures from foil and casting strips—this would be an ideal concretization of hope and comfort.

Creating someone who could watch over them, who could offer advice, was comforting and engaging. The girls were invested in and excited about their creations. Like the Phoenix rising from its own ashes, their angels became a symbol of renewed hope. Wings were made, figures were molded, and colors were painted on. Once the angels were completed, we began an intermodal exploration of these creatures. The girls were asked to tell each other the "creation story" of their angel. Using myth and storytelling, we listened to the stories of the angels they had created: " 'Hope' was born from the blowing of the wind," "My angel was born from the tears of a god." The following week, we returned to the angels; this time, we listened to the messages they had to give to us. The directive was to write a letter in the voice of the angel to yourself: What advice do you have to give? What are you guarding your maker from? What message do you want to give to the community as a whole? The girls then read their letters aloud to one another. They were encouraged to use feeling in their voices and gestures with their bodies to convey the messages. These messages were later placed on large strips as background to the wall under the ceiling from where the angels hung as an installation art piece.

Expressive Therapy in Individual Adult Psychotherapy

Jim is a 45-year-old self-employed accountant whom I've seen for individual psychotherapy at a small urban mental health center for 2 years. Jim came to therapy for help with his depression. Jim has had one psychiatric hospitalization for symptoms of paranoid schizophrenia, but minimizes the severity of his illness. Instead, Jim tends to focus on his need for help managing the posttraumatic stress symptoms he feels from a car accident he was in several years ago. In addition, he lives alone, has had no significant relationships (although he expresses an interest in dating women), and has a difficult relationship with his family who live about 30 miles away.

During one of our earliest sessions, Jim began by saying he had so many things to talk about he didn't know where to begin. He was distressed, unfocused, and disquieted. I invited Jim to look around the room and to find objects that represented the areas in his life he would like to explore. He chose a teapot to represent the sense of home and hospitality he wished to create in his small apartment; he chose a small statue of a figure thinking to represent his mental health issues; he chose a light yellow scarf to represent the femininity of the woman he would like to meet; he chose the phone to represent his business and work life. He was encouraged to intentionally place these objects on the floor of the room, in relation to one another, as close or as far as he felt they were in importance and proximity to one another. He worked quietly, with focus, investing energy and feeling into the act of arranging. He spoke about each object, remarking on how each object really seemed to "fit" its symbolic function.

After he had finished his arrangement, Jim was encouraged to stand in to the place of each one, to use sound, movement, enactment, and his body to explore the central message or question in each area. Despite a bit of initial discomfort with the "play acting," Jim quickly became excited by the sense of freedom he felt in the role of the "other." He was encouraged to give each position a voice, to speak from an "I" position—to use the psychodramatic technique of role reversal with each object (Leveton, 1977). Placing the hand of one arm on his hip and making the other arm a spout, he leaned over and hummed: "I pour warm tea. I am a server. I soothe and comfort Jim when he is having trouble sleeping at night." He waved the scarf gently in the air around him: "I am a pretty woman. I am a potential girlfriend. I am nice." He picked up the receiver on the phone and made a ringing noise: "Brrrrnggg . . . brrrrnggg. . . . "

"I'm not working enough," Jim said, suddenly out of role. "I'm worried about money. I really need to be able to focus more so that I can work even a couple of hours a day. I've been very unfocused with work." "I am confusion, I am paranoia." Jim took the role of the figure that represented his mental illness. For the first time in our sessions, Jim was able to tell me about his illness. He talked about his hospitalization and the impact that his illness has had on his ability to work and sustain focus. He was relieved and calm when he left the session.

Working in the role of the "other," allowing his imagination to lead him to the depth of his feelings, giving voice to aspects of his longing that had been split off and projected on others, were all possible through the use of the arts and through amplification via the intermodal process. Over the next several months, Jim and I were able to use his enactments as the touchstone from which we explored the various issues in his life. The energy of the images continued to live in our space. One by one we were able to call them back into the room, and through further imaginative encounters continue to explore their significance for Jim.

CONCLUSION

The combined use of the arts for healing is not a new phenomenon, but has been indigenous to cultures for centuries. It is time that intermodalists develop a voice in modern society. The most recent writings on expressive arts therapy have been theoretical, with the clinical examples often arising from students and workshop participants. The development of techniques of intermodality, of methods of integrated arts inquiry, and of multimodal assessment tools is necessary if we are to take our place as the "specialists" that we have become. More expressive therapists need to write about specific clinical examples of integrated arts therapy process in treatment with special needs populations. Questions need to be raised about the best time and place for an integrated arts process over a single-modal approach. When is an expressive arts therapy approach more useful? When is it less useful? How does the intermodalist decide when to transfer modalities? What is the best training for the expressive arts therapist? As these questions and methods become more explicit, expressive arts therapy can continue to solidify itself as the effective practice it's destined to become.

REFERENCES

Agell, G. (1982). Great debate: The place of art in art therapy: Art therapy or arts therapy? *American Journal of Art Therapy, 21*, 121–122.
Aldridge, D., Brandt, G., & Wohler, D. (1990). Toward a common language among the creative arts therapies. *Arts in Psychotherapy, 17*, 189–195.

Allen, J. (1993). Dissociative processes: Theoretical underpinnings of a working model for clinicians and patient. *Bulletin of the Menninger Clinic, 57*(3), 287–309.

Atkins, S. (2002). *Expressive arts therapy: Creative process in art and life.* Boone, NC: Parkway.

Blatner, A. (1992). Theoretical principles underlying creative arts therapies. *Arts in Psychotherapy, 18,* 405–409.

Fleshman, B., & Fryrear, J. L. (1981). *The arts in therapy.* Chicago: Nelson-Hall.

Gendlin, E. (1981). *Focusing* (2nd ed.). New York: Bantam Books.

Goren-Bar, A. (1994). Three self theories (H. Kohut, D. Stern, C. Bollas) applied to intermodal expressive therapy. *Dissertation Abstracts International, 55*(11–B), 506B. (UMI No. 9509282)

Goren-Bar, A. (1997). The "creation-axis" in expressive therapies. *Arts in Psychotherapy, 24*(5), 411–418.

Grenadier, S. (1995). The place wherein truth lies: An expressive therapy perspective on trauma, innocence and human nature. *Arts in Psychotherapy, 22*(5), 393–402.

Johnson, D. R. (1984). Establishing the creative arts therapies as an independent profession. *Arts in Psychotherapy, 11*(3), 209–212.

Johnson, D. R. (1985). Envisioning the link among the creative arts therapies. *Arts in Psychotherapy, 12*(4), 233–238.

Johnson, D. R. (1987). The role of the creative arts therapies in the diagnosis and treatment of psychological trauma. *Arts in Psychotherapy, 14*(1), 7–13.

Johnson, D. R. (1998). On the therapeutic action of the creative arts therapies: The psychodynamic model. *Arts in Psychotherapy, 25*(2), 85–99.

Johnson, D. R. (1999). *Essays on the creative arts therapies: Imaging a birth of a profession.* Springfield, IL: Thomas.

Knill, P. J. (1978). *Intermodal learning in education and therapy.* Cambridge, MA: Lesley College Arts Institute.

Knill, P. J. (1994). Multiplicity as a tradition: Theories for interdisciplinary arts therapies—An overview. *Arts in Psychotherapy, 21*(5), 319–328.

Knill, P. J., Barba, H. N., & Fuchs, M. N. (1995). *Minstrels of soul: Intermodal expressive therapy.* Toronto: Palmerston Press.

Lampropoulos, G. K. (2000). Evolving psychotherapy integration: Eclectic selection and prescriptive applications of common factors in therapy. *Psychotherapy: Theory, Research, Practice, Training, 37*(4), 285–297.

Langer, S. (1953). *Feeling and form.* New York: Scribner's.

Leveton, E. (1977). *Psychodrama for the timid clinician.* New York: Springer.

Levick, M. (1980). Response to Connie E. Naitove—"Creative arts therapist: Jack of all trades or master of one?" *Arts in Psychotherapy, 7*(4), 261–263.

Levine, E. (1995). *Tending the fire: Studies in art, therapy, and creativity.* Toronto: Palmerston Press/EGS Press.

Levine, S. K. (1992). *Poiesis: The language of psychology and the speech of the soul.* Toronto: Palmerston Press/Kingsley.

Levine, S. K., & Levine, E. G. (Eds.). (1999). *Foundations of expressive arts therapy: Theoretical and clinical perspectives*. London: Kingsley.

Lusebrink, V. B. (1992). A systems oriented approach to the expressive therapies: The expressive therapies continuum. *Arts in Psychotherapy, 18*(5), 39–403.

McNiff, S. (1979). From shamanism to art therapy. *Arts in Psychotherapy, 6*(3), 155–161.

McNiff, S. (1981). *The arts and psychotherapy*. Springfield, IL: Thomas.

McNiff, S. (1982). Great debate: The place of art in art therapy: Working with everything we have. *American Journal of Art Therapy, 21*(4), 122–123.

McNiff, S. (1986). *Educating the creative arts therapist: A profile of the profession*. Springfield, IL: Thomas.

McNiff, S. (1987). Pantheon of creative arts therapies: An integrative perspective. *Journal of Integrative and Eclectic Psychotherapy, 6*(3), 259–281.

McNiff, S. (1988). The shaman within. *Arts in Psychotherapy, 15*(4), 285–291.

McNiff, S. (1992). *Art as medicine: Creating a therapy of the imagination*. Boston: Shambhala.

McNiff, S. (1998). Review of J. Chodorow's *Jung on active imagination*. *Art Therapy: Journal of the American Art Therapy Association, 15*(4), 269–272.

McNiff, S. (2000). Pandora's gift: The use of imagination and all of the arts in therapy. In J. A. Rubin (Ed.), *Approaches to art therapy: Theory and technique* (2nd ed., pp. 318–325). Philadelphia: Brunner-Routledge.

Naitove, C. E. (1980). Creative arts therapist: Jack of all trades or master of one? *Arts in Psychotherapy, 7*(4), 253–259.

Robbins, A. (1980). *Expressive therapy: A creative arts approach to depth-oriented treatment*. New York: Human Sciences Press.

Robbins, A. (1985). Working towards the establishment of creative arts therapies as an independent profession. *Arts in Psychotherapy, 12*(2), 67–70.

Robbins, A. (1988). A psychoaesthetic perspective on creative arts therapy and training. *Arts in Psychotherapy, 15*(2), 95–100.

Rogers, N. (1993). *The creative connection: Expressive arts as healing*. Palo Alto, CA: Science and Behavior Books.

Shakur, T. (1995). So many tears. On *Me against the world* [CD]. New York: Amaru/Jive Records.

Smeijsters, H. (1993). Music therapy in the Netherlands. In C. D. Maranto, *Music therapy: International perspectives* (pp. 385–421). Pipersville, PA: Jeffrey Books. (Also found at *www.gironet.nl/home/kjk97/mtnleng.htm*)

Speiser, P. (1996). The development of an expressive arts therapist as a paradigm for the development of a field. Unpublished doctoral dissertation, Union Institute, 1996. (*Dissertation Abstracts International, 57*(5–B), 3425)

van der Kolk, B., & van der Hart, O. (1991). The intrusive past: The flexibility of memory and the engraving of trauma. *American Imago, 48,* 425–454.

Weston, D. (1994). Toward an integrative model of affect regulation: Applications to social-psychological research. *Journal of Personality, 62*(4), 641–667.

Wiener, D. (Ed.). (1999). *Beyond talk therapy: Using movement and expressive techniques in clinical practice.* Washington, DC: American Psychological Association.

Wiener, D., & Oxford, L. (Eds.). (2003). *Action therapy with families and groups: Using creative arts improvisation in clinical practice.* Washington, DC: American Psychological Association.

Winnicott, D. W. (1971). *Playing and reality.* London and New York: Routledge.

ॐ Appendix

Professional Organizations

American Art Therapy Association
1202 Allanson Road
Mundelein, IL 60060-3808
Phone: 888-290-0878 or 847-949-6064
Fax: 847-566-4580
E-mail: *info@arttherapy.org*
Website: *www.arttherapy.org*

The AATA is a national association dedicated to the belief that the creative process involved in the making of art is healing and life-enhancing. Founded in 1969, the AATA is a not-for-profit organization of professionals and students that has established standards for art therapy education, ethics, and practice.

American Counseling Association
Association for Creativity in Counseling Division
5999 Stevenson Avenue
Alexandria, VA 22304
Phone: 800-347-6647
Fax: 800-473-2329
Website: *www.counseling.org*

The ACA is a not-for-profit professional and educational organization that is dedicated to the growth and enhancement of the counseling profession. Founded in 1952, the ACA is the world's largest association exclusively representing professional counselors in various practice settings. The Association for Creativity in Counseling was established in 2004 and provides a forum for research, education, and scholarly exchange on the use of creative modalities in clinical work.

211

American Dance Therapy Association
2000 Century Plaza, Suite 108
10632 Little Patuxent Parkway
Columbia, MD 21044
Fax: 410-997-4048
Website: *www.adta.org*

Founded in 1966, the ADTA works to establish high standards of professional education and competence in the field of dance/movement therapy. It stimulates communication among dance/movement therapists and members of allied professions.

American Music Therapy Association
8455 Colesville Road, Suite 1000
Silver Spring, MD 20910
Phone: 301-589-3300
Fax: 301-589-5175
Website: *www.musictherapy.org*

Founded in 1998, the AMTA's purpose is the progressive development of the therapeutic use of music in rehabilitation, special education, and community settings. The AMTA is committed to the advancement of education, training, professional standards, credentials, and research in support of the music therapy profession.

American Society of Group Psychotherapy and Psychodrama
Website: *www.asgpp.org*

Founded in 1942 by J. L. Moreno, MD, the ASGPP fosters national and international cooperation among all who are concerned with the theory and practice of psychodrama, sociometry, and group psychotherapy. It works to promote application of theories, dissemination of information, and publication of research, and to encourage and promote professional training and a code of professional standards in these fields.

British Association of Play Therapists
31 Cedar Drive
Keynsham, Bristol, England BS31 2TY
Phone and fax: 01179 860390
E-mail: *info@bapt.uk.com*
Website: *www.bapt.info*

The BAPT is the professional association that governs play therapy in Great Britain, including training, standards, practice, and the development of the profession.

Canadian Association for Child and Play Therapy
2 Bloor Street West, #100
Toronto, Ontario, Canada M4W 3E2
Phone: 800-361-3951 (voicemail only) or 519-524-5990
Fax: 519-524-6537
E-mail: *cacpt@hurontel.on.ca*
Website: *www.cacpt.com*

The CACPT promotes the understanding and value of play therapy, high standards of professional and ethical practice, and professional training and current research in the field.

International Expressive Arts Therapy Association
P.O. Box 320399
San Francisco, CA 94132
Phone: 415-522-8959
Website: *www.ieata.org*

The IETA is a nonprofit organization that provides ongoing local and global information exchange within the expressive arts field for artists, educators, therapists, and other creative-minded individuals.

International Society for Sandplay Therapy
Website: *www.sandplayusa.org*

The ISST is a nonprofit association formed in 1985 to continue the development of sandplay therapy as formulated by founder Dora M. Kalff. With chapters in Canada, Germany, Great Britain, Israel, Italy, Japan, Switzerland, and the United States, it provides a meeting ground for the international exchange of knowledge and experience in sandplay.

National Association for Drama Therapy
15 Post Side Lane
Pittsford, NY 14534
Phone: 585-381-5618
Fax: 585-383-1474
E-mail: *answers@nadt.org*
Website: *www.nadt.org*

The NADT is a nonprofit association incorporated in 1979 to establish and uphold high standards of professional competence and ethics among drama therapists; to develop criteria for training and registration; to sponsor publications and conferences; and to promote the profession of drama therapy through information and advocacy.

National Association for Poetry Therapy
Marge Silberling, Administrator
16861 SW 6th Street
Pembroke Pines, FL 33027
Phone: 866-844-NAPT or 954-499-4333
Fax: 954-499-4324
Website: *www.poetrytherapy.org*

The NAPT is a community of healers and lovers of words and language who work in diverse settings where people deal with personal and communal pain and the search for growth. Its members include psychotherapists, poets, educators, physicians, clergy, artists, dramatists, musicians, and writers.

Sandplay Therapists of America
P.O. Box 4847
Walnut Creek, CA 94596
Phone: 925-825-9277
E-mail: *sta@sandplay.org*
Website: *www.sandplayusa.org/stainfo.html*

STA is a nonprofit organization established to train, support, and promote professional development in sandplay therapy in the tradition of Dora Kalff as based on the theories of C. G. Jung.

Index

"f" following a page number indicates a figure; "t" following a page number indicates a table.